The Psychological Impact of Chronic Illness: A Practical Guide for Primary Care Physicians

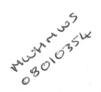

The Psychological Impact of Acute and Chronic Illness:

Tamara McClintock Greenberg, PsyD, MS
San Francisco, CA

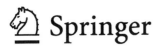 Springer

Tamara McClintock Greenberg, Psy.D., M.S.
University of California, San Francisco
Langley Porter Psychiatric Institute
San Francisco, CA 94143
Private Practice, San Francisco

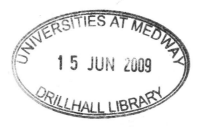

Library of Congress Control Number: 2006925258

ISBN-10: 0-387-33682-6   e-ISBN-10: 0-387-38298-4
ISBN-13: 978-0-387-33682-4   e-ISBN-13: 978-0-387-38298-2

Printed on acid-free paper.

9 8 7 6 5 4 3 2 1

springer.com

*This book is dedicated to all of the patients who have taught me,
through their courageous struggles with illness, about the impact and
meaning of the diseases that plague us.*

T. M. G.

FOREWORD

In the following pages, Dr. Greenberg delineates the complex forces at play within patients who are newly ill or disabled, within physicians who do their best to guide patients through those debilities, and in the interaction that patient–physician dyads perform thousands of times daily to try to make sense of the patient's plight.

As a physician and medical educator who thinks about how to enhance communication between patients and physicians, I often view communication challenges as arising from divergent cultural experiences. Each patient has a unique method of experiencing, deriving meaning from, and coping with a new or chronic illness. This approach is necessarily filtered through the patient's family and social contexts and the patient's current living situation.

Physicians, too, bring psychosocial upbringing and current social context into their clinical practice settings. We have also been inculcated into a medical culture that takes its bright, impressionable, idealistic young and shapes them, sometimes brutally, into diagnosticians and proceduralists. We are just now beginning to understand the many components of the "hidden curriculum" of many medical schools – unspoken but powerful influences in training that undercut the humanity of trainees and turn them into poorer communicators than when they first started.

The challenge is to achieve and prioritize connection, both in medical education and in practice. Many of my procedure-based colleagues achieve this nonverbally, by fixing a problem, and many patients deeply appreciate their outcomes. An equally powerful connection forms through empathic witnessing of a patient's situation, even if we cannot fully understand all that a patient might be undergoing. In addition, research suggests that the presence of an empathic statement in both medical and surgical settings can *decrease* the length of an outpatient encounter. Presumably, as clinicians share that they understand what a patient might be undergoing, the patient leaves more satisfied. This outcome is clearly desirable for patients, physicians, and health care systems.

The other day, I saw Mr. A, elderly in years but still sprightly. When I first met him, about four years ago, I found his communication style somewhat challenging. He would flit from subject to subject, most of which were nonmedical and which I deemed unimportant. He told me about classes he took at the local community college on spirituality and love. He told me of his son, his divorce, and continuing loving relationship with his ex-wife, his present friendships, and his continued sexual escapades, both consensual and individual. He showed me photos of his artwork and of himself when he was younger. Each time he left the office, I knew I was missing his point: somehow he was trying to tell me something, but I was too dense, too distracted, and mostly too uninterested to figure it out. Anyway, it was onward immediately to the next patient, so I never stopped to think about it.

Over time he had to have a total knee replacement, then a coronary bypass, and, most recently, urgent surgery for a humeral fracture suffered in a fall. Through these major procedures, Mr. A was sunny, upbeat, and completely (and a bit maddeningly) insistent on continuing to tell me tangential stories.

So when I saw him on my schedule the other day, I was expecting more of the same. Instead, in walked a rather dour man dressed in gray and black, when I'd come to expect vibrant multiple colors. At once I knew that Mr. A had reached the limits of his substantial coping ability. Three successive surgical procedures and rehabilitation processes had finally taken their toll. He could neither walk nor lift his dominant arm without pain, and he began to despair that he would never regain full function. He'd stopped his numerous activities, was eating and sleeping poorly, clearly had low energy, and could not concentrate. Though he vehemently denied suicidal ideation. When I asked him, "Do you have any guilt?", he instantly became tearful. He spoke of how he was re-evaluating his life and felt that he'd been terribly selfish with his ex-wife; maybe if he'd treated her better, they'd still be together. The loneliness was palpable. Now I understood the

the *person*, not the organism. In response, I'd left his gift unopened on my stoop, wondering if it would go away.

Now that I could understand more about my own resistance to Mr. A's stories, I found myself more fully appreciating him. As a doctor I often feel compelled, as Dr. Greenberg notes in Chapter 2, to action. Though Mr. A and I went through the obligatory discussion about antidepressants (see Chapter 5), I felt an important need just to be in the same space as he. Somewhere, deep inside, I was saying to myself, "Don't just do something, be there."

By the end of the visit, Mr. A felt compelled to quote a poem of Edna St. Vincent Millay called 'Love Is Not All.' Though I'm generally not a "poetry person," by his ability to reach through his depression into himself and share a piece of his passion with me, I knew that my low-tech intervention of empathic witnessing had succeeded.

Calvin Chou, MD, PhD
Associate Professor of Clinical Medicine
University of California, San Francisco

FOREWORD

This is a particularly challenging time in medicine. While our scientific knowledge is rapidly expanding, both patient and clinician satisfaction with our health care system is declining. Students enter medical school with strong humanistic and ethical ideals. Over the four years, they assimilate more knowledge than they knew possible. They are then faced with several years of residency when they must continue to acquire knowledge and skills while providing direct patient care. Given the enormity of this task, our education and health care systems encourage a primary focus on the traditional, evidence-based science of medicine. The psychology of illness is either assumed to be self-evident or is left to the purview of mental health professionals. This is not a realistic approach and not what most of us desire from our physicians.

As individuals, nobody teaches us how to think about and respond to illness. Although virtually all medical schools now teach some form of the psychology of illness, most students attend first to the "hard" science courses, fitting in the "less scientific" courses as time permits. Residents quickly learn the frustration that comes from dealing only with the illness when they see Mrs. Smith back for her ninth admission in three months with the exact same symptoms. It's as though they have the know-how to pull a car out of a skid, can tell people in detail how to respond, and then have to watch person after person go into a skid. Clearly, something more is needed.

Dr. Greenberg examines the history of illness and psychology, giving the reader a context for current beliefs and practices in Western medicine. It is generally acknowledged that certain illnesses, like asthma, have a psychosomatic component. Unfortunately, many people think this means the illness is in the sufferer's head, that the symptoms are not real. Studies clearly show that mood state affects the outcome of a variety of illnesses, like coronary artery disease. Most physicians continue to focus on the hard facts: tests, treatments, etc. Most patients, however, care most about their ability to function and engage in their lives.

Bringing her years of work as an astute and respected clinician, educator, and colleague, Dr. Greenberg demystifies patients' psychological needs, giving the reader an understanding of and an approach to caring for the entire patient. We all have different coping strategies, roles, relationships, and predisposition to mental illness that are brought to bear in dealing with illness, which is among the most stressful tasks of living. As clinicians, we interact with the illness and the patient before us, as well as with their entire history, family, culture, and level of trust of the medical establishment. Although referral to a mental health practitioner in conjunction with ongoing primary care is sometimes the answer, it is neither possible nor desirable in all instances. Dr. Greenberg demonstrates the synthesis of medical and psychological approaches into a coherent treatment approach.

This wonderful book is a must-read for all clinicians. Use it repeatedly as a reference; both you and your patients will benefit greatly.

Lee Jones, MD
Associate Dean for Student Affairs
Professor, Department of Psychiatry
UTHSC San Antonio

PREFACE

Medicine is a rapidly changing field. The many variables in the practice of modern medicine—the influence of technology on medicine, HMOs, the complicated psychological dynamics that patients bring to physicians, the changes in pharmacological treatments for mental disorders, and family dynamics and interactions—all make the practice of medicine difficult and complicated. The demands on physicians are unprecedented. Patient expectations are increasing and, as the population ages, are likely only to continue to increase. These changes will probably intensify the demands placed on physicians. Changes in the population of patients seen in today's medical offices require an increase in flexibility, as well as sensitivity, which makes the practice of medicine more interesting, and also more demanding, than ever before. I hope that this book can help ease the burden on physicians.

The purpose of this book is to help clinicians understand the normative as well as maladaptive reactions to illness. It is intended for primary care physicians, who as front-line clinicians provide the majority of medical as well as mental health treatments for a large number of patients in the general population. Specialist physicians may also benefit from the explanations provided in this book on the psychological dynamics of illness, as they, too, are confronted with patients for whom coping with illness is a major factor in treatment. Providers of psychological services who deal with medical patients may also find this book useful because it normalizes a lot of the issues in medical patients that some mental health clinicians may be tempted to pathologize.

One of the major changes in the current practice of medicine is related to the work of primary care physicians as mental health practitioners. Primary care clinicians prescribe more antidepressants than any other prescribers, and the field of psychotropic medication has changed and expanded in recent years with an increasing array of medication choices for patients with anxiety and depression. Chapter 5 attempts to decode many of the issues that primary physicians face when prescribing antidepressants and anxiolytics for patients and to address the potential pitfalls (i.e., medication interactions) that can occur when prescribing for patients with medical problems. Although physicians can pharmacologically treat a number of mental health problems, the need for a mental health presence with medical patients is increasing. Yet many physicians feel confused about how to refer patients for mental health treatment. Chapter 9 should help reduce the difficulty many physicians face when trying to refer patients for mental health treatment. Other chapters in this book are designed to help physicians understand the complicated and sometimes confusing reactions (e.g., helplessness or noncompliance) patients and their families have in response to serious illness.

I see patients in acute hospital settings and nursing homes, as well as in my outpatient private practice. I have been fortunate to work with the University of California, San Francisco, medical hospitals and clinics since 1997. This work started with a cardiothoracic surgeon, David Jablons, MD; I saw patients with thoracic malignancies in an outpatient clinic. I then began seeing patients who had a variety of physical disorders in Mt. Zion Hospital and then in the UCSF hospitals. Today I tend to see a limited number of hospital patients and continue to have relationships with certain UCSF faculty practice groups and to provide pre- and postoperative evaluations, pretransplant evaluations, and ongoing treatment for medical patients. I also have been fortunate to work with medical students in the UCSF Medical School, who continually educate me regarding the rigors of medical education and practice.

There are a number of colleagues who generously offered their time and expertise to read chapters and provide feedback regarding the concepts discussed in this book. Thanks to Greg Berman, MD; Peter Carnachan, PhD; Bart Magee, PhD; Kathleen Regan, MSN, NP; Anne O'Crowley, PhD; Annie Sweetnam, PhD; Maxine Papadakis, MD; Michael Guy Thompson, PhD; and Steve Tulkin, PhD, MS.

I am thankful to Rob Albano, my senior editor at Springer, who helped me translate the initial ideas for this book into a practical form and to clarify how this book might be most useful for physicians. I also appreciate the

valuable, Andrew was able to offer the clinician's perspective on the realities of patient care and medical practice in today's complicated world.

I am indebted to the patients who over the years have influenced my thinking about psychological responses to illness. It is through their courage, honesty, and insights that I developed a real and nonacademic understanding of the impact of acute and chronic illness. It is ultimately for them that this book was written, and it would have been impossible without their trust in me as a clinician. Though all cases in this book are based on actual patient encounters, identifying information has been altered to protect confidentiality and disguise identity.

Tamara McClintock Greenberg, PsyD, MS
San Francisco, CA

CONTENTS

1

"It is more important to know what kind of patient has the disease than what kind of disease the patient has."

—Sir William Olser

The interaction of the mind and the body has been of interest to many physicians, philosophers, and more recently psychologists, for hundreds of years. In recent years there has been increasing interest regarding how emotional factors, which include some psychiatric illnesses, coping skills, emotional states, and personality traits, impact physical health. Research regarding emotional factors and illness has demonstrated powerful links between the mind and the body. This chapter will review selected medical and psychological research in this area and will discuss possible mechanisms to explain these associations.

Medical and psychological researchers and clinicians have long known that psychological problems can manifest themselves physically (e.g., through psychosomatic disorders). More recently, there has been an increased understanding that not only is the impact of emotional coping important in persons who are already ill, but also that emotional states (including depression, anxiety, and hostility) are associated with the development of certain illness. Although the culture of Western medicine (which will be discussed further in Chapter 2) has taught us that the mind and the body are separate, there is mounting evidence that the mind and body are symbiotic and that strong interactions between the two exist.

There are two important general areas of research related to interactions between emotional and physical functioning. The first area deals with certain emotional states and their role in the development or exacerbation of certain illnesses. The second major area I will address is the impact of coping on illness. The discussion on coping will deal with day-to-day responses to stressful events, attitudes, perceptions, and the use of religion and social support. Although there are certainly similarities between emotional states and coping, the coping research tends to focus on responses of persons assessed to be psychologically (and sometimes physically) healthy. Another interesting distinction between these two areas of concentration is that the research on emotional states and illness is often found in major medical journals. The research on coping is found more often in psychological journals. This difference may reflect differences in the fields of medicine and psychology in terms of what is regarded as "clinically significant" research. Further, the research on coping often addresses the impact of thoughts and attitudes that are present in most of us. The subjects of research on emotional states, in contrast, tend to be persons with difficulty in coping and resulting depression or intense anxiety. Additionally, the research on emotions focuses on personality traits such as hostility, cynicism, and mistrust that are not related to coping per se, but dramatically impact psychological processes. After presenting the research on emotional states and coping, I will discuss areas of research that do not seem to fit the category of either emotional states or coping. These areas include the large volume of research on stress, racial and economic disparities in health care, and the impact of child abuse on physical functioning.

DEPRESSION

Most, if not all, health care providers are aware of the high incidence of depression. Recent statistics from the American Psychological Association report that in the United States depression occurs in one out of five women and in about one out of ten men at some point in the lifespan.[1] Because of its prevalence, depression is thought by many to be a major cause of disability worldwide for both young and older adults.

Medical patients are more likely to be depressed than persons without chronic medical conditions, and the number of chronic medical conditions is positively correlated with an increased risk of depression.[2]

this research did not gain momentum until the mid-1990s.

Perhaps the most replicated and striking research related to depression and the development of medical problems is that depression has been found to play a role in the development of cardiovascular disease. Depression has been found to predict some forms of heart disease, which is the leading cause of death in the United States. Some of the earlier research in this area found that in persons who had pre-existing heart disease, depression predicted a poorer prognosis. For example, depression was found to independently predict a second myocardial infarction (MI) in patients who have already had a myocardial infarction.[3] Additionally, depression also predicts poorer survival among patients with coronary artery disease (CAD) and congestive heart failure (CHF).[4,5] Although much of the depression/heart disease research has suggested that people who are already ill and depressed live shorter lifespans, there is also evidence that major depression and depressive symptoms are associated with a first MI.[6–8] Although so far I have been describing research in which subjects were diagnosed with major depressive disorder (in most cases based on *Diagnostic and Statistical Manual of Mental Disorders* criteria), even persons who have a few symptoms of depression (minimal depressive symptoms as measured by the Beck Depression Inventory) and do not meet criteria for major depressive disorder are at increased risk for a subsequent myocardial infarction if they already have heart disease.[9] It should be mentioned that while earlier research focused primarily on men, due the increased prevalence of heart disease, similar findings have emerged in women.

Depression leads to poorer outcomes in both the elderly as well as medical inpatients. Patients who are both elderly and hospitalized are at greater risk of experiencing the negative impact of depression. Depression predicts greater physical decline among the elderly. Among hospital inpatients with a variety of illnesses, depressed mood was an independent risk factor for mortality.[10,11] Some of the research on depression has assessed the risk of depression as compared with other risk factors. For example, a study of elderly women found that the risk of death due from depression was as significant as risks from smoking, high cholesterol, obesity, and diabetes.[12]

The research on depression and later development of cancer has yielded less consistent results than other research on depression and illness. Many confounding variables (e.g., the varying pathophysiology of different types of cancer, the effects of some cancers on the endocrine system, mood symptoms in response to chemotaxic agents, etc.) make studying associations between depression and cancer difficult. However, reviews of the literature and meta-analyses have found weak associations between depression and the development of cancer and slightly stronger associations between depression and the progression of cancer.[13–15] Additionally, although there have been inconsistent results, at least two studies have found associations between chronic depression and the development of breast cancer.[16,17] One difficulty in the cancer/depression research is that chronicity of depression is not always studied, and the measures of depression differ in many studies. A 2003 article by David Spiegel and Janine Giese-Davis, who are leading experts in this field, suggested that because of the inconsistent findings and methodological problems assessing depression in this patient population, there is only weak evidence linking depression and development of cancer, but that there is likely stronger evidence of an association between depression and cancer progression and shorter survival time.[18] These authors note, however, that the methodological problems such as not assessing chronic depression may obscure current interpretations of this research. Additionally, the physical effects of cancer can mimic neurovegetative signs of depression, thus further complicating the interpretation of research. Perhaps as more researchers study chronic depression, which could potentially cause alterations in immune functioning over time, we will have a clearer understanding of a depression and cancer association.

Emerging research links depression and loss of bone density. Studies indicate that in both young and perimenopausal women, depression is associated with an increased risk of osteoporosis.[19,20] One of these studies found an increased risk of bone density loss in women with both depression and borderline personality disorder.[20] There is also evidence that depression is also associated with decreased bone mineral density in men.[21,22]

In a nationally representative sample of men and women, depression was predictive of hip fracture even after controlling for other risk factors.[23]

depression. Anxiety is also difficult to study due to the differences between trait anxiety (meaning that some people are always worried and nervous) and state anxiety, which involves the anxiety that emerges in all of us in day-to-day life. Indeed, anxiety is intimately connected with the sympathetic nervous system and the "fight/flight" response. Without anxiety, humans could not have evolved as successfully as we have; we need anxiety for our survival. Despite this, we all know persons for whom anxiety is more than just normative. Persons like this tend to panic over small things; they worry constantly, and some anxious people have the effect of making others around them anxious as well.

Despite the difficulties of studying anxiety, research has emerged that implicates the negative impact of certain kinds of anxiety. Reviews of the literature suggest that patients with panic disorder as well as chronic anxiety have higher rates of hypertension, CAD, and heart disease.[24,25] It should be noted that another recent literature review cited that the impact of anxiety and the development of heart disease as well as anxiety and the progression of heart disease have been inconsistent, with about half of studies showing significant associations in healthy samples and about one-third of studies showing associations in patients with known heart disease.[26] Additionally, anxiety, especially phobic anxiety, has long been anecdotally associated with sudden cardiac death, and this finding is suggested in empirical studies as well.[27,28]

HOSTILITY

Research on hostility actually has roots in the old "Type A" research that took place in the 1970s.[29] Type A is a construct that was developed following the observation that persons with heart disease tended to be impatient, hard-driving, and aggressive men who worked too much. While the Type A research yielded a lot of popular interest in the concept that still exists today (I frequently hear patients describe themselves or others as "Type A"), there is not much statistical validity to the cluster of traits describing Type A. In other words, the concept of Type A did not have enough traits that were similar to one another to form a concept that made sense and that fit the profile of heart patients. However, research has shown that anger and hostility are key traits within the Type A construct and that these traits are present in some patients with cardiovascular disease. As these traits were studied more intensely, it was found that the kind of anger and hostility manifested in some patients with cardiovascular disease reflected cynical mistrust. The questions on the Cook-Medley Hostility Scale, which is frequently used to measure hostility, demonstrate the type of hostility I am describing.[30] Some items on this instrument are (respondents answer true or false): "I tend to be on my guard with people who are more friendly than I expected," "I have often felt that strangers were looking at me critically," "I have at times had to be rough with people who were rude to me," and "I have often met people who were supposed to be experts who were no better than I." Respondents who answer true to these types of questions are likely to be high in hostility as well as cynical mistrust.

Reviews of several studies, including ten prospective studies found that trait hostility is related to an increased risk of developing heart disease, although the role of hostility in persons who have established heart disease is less clear.[31–33] Further, a tendency to express anger has been implicated as a potential trigger for MI.[34] It should be noted that some researchers have questioned the strength of these associations in terms of their practical applicability.[32] Nevertheless, much of the research suggests a trend in the direction in terms of hostility's contribution to heart disease.

One could imagine that persons high in hostility and cynical mistrust might have difficulties in social relationships. Persons who are hostile in the way described above would likely approach relationships in a suspicious way, which would make it difficult to establish and maintain closeness. There is evidence that persons who are hostile have difficulty accessing social support. The impact of hostility and cynicism is problematic in terms of how it limits possible benefit from social support (We will see shortly that social support plays a major role in morbidity and

Table 1. Medical effects of emotional states

Emotional state	Associations
Depression	MI (both subsequent and first)
	CAD
	Heart disease
Hostility/cynicism	Coronary calcification
	Atherosclerosis
	Hypertension
	Heart disease

mortality in some patient populations), as cynical people have difficulty making use of the social support available to them.[35,36]

Also, an excellent prospective study with young adults found that trait hostility and cynical distrust is predictive of increased coronary calcification after adjusting for age, demographic, and lifestyle variables.[37] What is fascinating about this study is that it involved young men and women (ages eighteen to thirty) who were healthy, but over the ten years that the study took place these people developed coronary calcification, an atherosclerotic precursor, if they had high levels of hostility and mistrust.

Table 1 summarizes the major research linking emotional states and illness.

COPING AND ILLNESS

Another aspect of the psychological/physical research looks at coping and its impact on quality of life, disease progression, morbidity, and mortality. This body of research is rooted largely in early studies by health psychology researchers, and it looks at the coping behaviors that often occur in the general population. I tend to think of this body of research as slightly more "positively" oriented. Much of the coping research has historically taken place in healthy young adults, although as more links between psychological and physical functioning are documented, more medical patients have been studied in regard to how they cope with illness. Some of the main research in this area involves benefits of social support, use of religion, attitudes of pessimism or optimism, and the extent to which patients feel control over aspects of their illness and treatment.

Social Support

Social support can be thought of as physical and emotional help that is available to us in our environment. There are wide variations in the availability of support to people at different times in their lives. As people get older, their social support network can dwindle; friends and spouses become ill or die, retirement changes social contacts, adult children become involved in their own lives, and so on. I often hear patients complain that as they become older, they have to work much harder at maintaining a network of close friends. As people get older, work becomes the main place for making friends. If one works in a job where there is limited access to co-workers it can be very difficult to find friends. (It used to be true that dating was difficult in these circumstances, but fortunately the Internet has made that easier.) People who do not have access to social contacts at their place of employment usually make friends through their children (especially when children are young) or religious associations. For some people, though, work is the main place where socializing takes place. In these individuals, retirement reduces social contacts and loneliness increases.

Almost everyone has heard stories that once a spouse dies, the other spouse is likely to die as well within a relatively short period of time. There is research to support this assumption.[38] One way to understand this finding is that there is an expected link between social support and depression. Social support buffers against the development of depression as well as against life stressors (which could include illness), and depressed mood can decrease the ability to access social support. Although depression and social isolation are interrelated, it has been found that for patients following acute MI, social isolation independently predicts mortality.[39–41]

In the general population, lacking social ties is associated with increases in mortality, and having social ties is linked with an increase in life-span.[42,43] It has also been demonstrated that individuals who lack social support have lower immune responses. In a study with healthy college students, students who reported fewer social supports and reported feeling lonely had a poorer immune response to the flu vaccine.[44] This reduction in antibody response lasted up to four months following administration of the flu shot.

dementia, Parkinson's disease, and rheumatoid arthritis, as well as increases in chronic pain-related disability.[45] This review also showed that although marriage has general protective health effects in both men and women, the increase in mortality from marriage is more robust in men and, interestingly, the effects of bad marriages appear to affect women more than men.

Religion

Recently, investigators have attempted to understand the impact of religion on coping with illness as well as its potential buffering effect against depression. There are difficulties in studying religion, however, because religion can be utilized to increase one's social support network, possibly confounding the findings in these studies. Many very religious patients I have seen have close social contacts through their religious organizations. Although this increase in social support may be one protective aspect of religion, persons who are religious often describe aspects of their faith that are not social. Praying, the sense of a personal relationship with God, and the sense of knowing what will happen to them when they die are all comforting to patients and may increase coping ability and reduce distress. Conversely, although religion can be comforting, there are some patients for whom religious beliefs seem to be unhelpful. These persons often report feeling abandoned by God, blaming God for their difficulties, or feeling that they are being punished for some wrongdoing in the past. Because of the different ways persons utilize religion, religious coping has been divided into two categories: positive religious coping and negative religious coping. Not surprisingly, positive religious coping is associated with fewer depressive symptoms and negative religious coping with more depressive symptoms. In a review of 147 studies examining the correlations between religion and depression, it was determined that positive religious coping is associated with fewer depressive symptoms, especially in times of stress.[46] This same review found that negative religious coping was associated with an increase of depressive symptoms. The use of religion has also been found to reduce distress and disability in end-stage pulmonary patients as well as to reduce anxiety in heart disease patients.[47,48]

There are also associations with religion and improved overall physical health.[49,50] One of these studies found that in Mexican Americans, religious attendance was associated with decreased mortality. Again, it is difficult to know the exact meaning of these studies in terms of which aspects of religion are protective (whether social support is a main factor or if there are other important variables), but nonetheless, the research in this area will likely yield interesting findings over the next several years.

Personality Factors

Although social support has been found to be beneficial to health, it is reasonable to assume that the importance of social support may vary among different people. For example, we all have seen patients who seem to have a wonderful support system: a loving spouse, caring children, a kind physician, and even a large network of friends, yet they do not seem to appreciate it much, may feel lonely or isolated or misunderstood, or may not seem to notice the kindness of those around them. I have learned a great deal about social support from meeting with young adults who have developed leukemia or lymphoma. Obviously this is a devastating and terrifying event for these young patients, but the wide range of responses that I see among these women and men continually strikes me. For example, some patients, although sad and scared, take up the challenge of their illness with remarkable courage and strength. They go through their treatment without incident and have good relationships with their health care providers. In sharp contrast, other patients become very angry. They resent everyone around them, are consumed with envy regarding those who are healthy, and tend to have negative relationships with the health care professionals who are trying to take care of them and with the family members who are trying to be supportive. Later chapters will identify some of the contributing dynamics in this group of patients. There is research evidence that not only do some personality traits impact the ability to access social support, but also some personality types have a harder time dealing with illness than oth

patients as being vulnerable to psychosomatic symptoms (and this is a correct assumption according to the research), people who experience a range of negative emotions may be vulnerable to "real" illnesses as well. One pathway to understanding this is that persons who are high in negative affect are less likely to perceive having social support available to them, even if they do have support around them.[51] Not only does negative trait affect interfere with the ability to access social support, but also there is evidence that negative affect correlates with altered immune responses. In one study with healthy adults, negative affect was associated with a lower antibody response to the hepatitis B vaccine.[52]

In persons who are ill, negativity is associated with a more rapid disease progression. For example, in men with HIV, negative expectations regarding the course of disease were associated with disease decline, including the onset of symptoms in previously asymptomatic patients.[53] Another aspect of negativity is pessimism. Pessimists not only tend to see the glass as half empty, they also tend to be harsh on themselves and often blame themselves for negative events. In elderly adults, a pessimistic attitude was associated with reductions in cell-mediated immunity.[54]

Another way of looking at negativity is to examine the impact of its opposite, what we might think of as positive coping styles, such as optimism. There is evidence that people with optimistic personalities have an easier time accessing social support, are more motivated to cope with illness in an active way, and are less prone to depression and hopelessness in the face of a stressful illness. Specifically, optimism is associated with faster recovery from coronary artery bypass surgery (CABG).[55] In this study, men who were optimists reported better quality of life six months and five years following surgery. Similar results have been found with women who underwent CABG.[56] Optimism is also associated with reports of less pain in patients with early-to-intermediate-stage rheumatoid arthritis (RA).[57]

An additional facet to optimism is "benefit finding" from the negative experiences one encounters in life, including illness. An example of this is a patient describing that although her struggle with cancer has been awful, the experience has helped her recognize her sense of purpose or to place greater value on the importance of her primary relationships. The construct of benefit finding has its roots in the trauma literature; since a serious medical illness is often traumatic, looking at its impact in persons with illness seems natural. Although the research is not overwhelming, finding benefit in one's illness does seem to have psychological and possibly physical implications. A study with breast cancer patients found that patients who were able to attribute some kind of benefit and meaning to their disease in the first year were in less distress five to eight years after diagnosis and reported fewer symptoms of depression.[58] A longitudinal study with HIV-positive gay men found that men who were able to find meaning through bereavement of a partner or a close friend had a slower rate of CD4 cell decline and had lower AIDS-related mortality at two to three years followup.[59]

Another aspect of coping with illness is the extent to which patients feel that they are active participants in their care and have a degree of control over their health-related outcome. We all know patients who react to their illness by being passive, probably due to a sense of helplessness. Research suggests that passivity is detrimental. For example, passive coping is a predictor of pain and depression in patients with RA.[60] In a longitudinal study of over 2,000 Dutch nationals who had a number of chronic diseases, including chronic obstructive pulmonary disease (COPD), heart disease, diabetes mellitus, and severe low back pain, an increased level of disability was associated with passive coping and a sense of not having any control over one's health.[61] In this study, death was a measure of disability, and the only psychological factor associated with mortality was a sense of control over one's health; those with a low sense of control had higher rates of mortality. Table 2 summarizes the research reviewed related to coping and health.

ADDITIONAL FACTORS

Although much of the research can be separated into emotional states and coping and its impact on illness, there are other factors that do not fit neatly into either category. The three remaining areas I will address are the

Table 2. Coping factors and medical effects

Coping factors	Associated medical effects
Lack of social support	All causes of mortality
	Mortality in heart disease
	Decreased distress, end-stage pulmonary patients
	Decreased anxiety in heart disease
Negative religious coping	Increased depression
Religious practices	Better physical health
	Decreased mortality
Negative trait affect	Less likely to benefit from social support
	Lower antibody response to hepatitis B vaccine
	More rapid disease decline in HIV-positive men
Pessimism	Reduced cell-mediated immunity (in the elderly)
Optimism	Faster recovery from CABG surgery
	Reduced pain in RA
Benefit finding	Reduced distress and depression in breast cancer
	Slower rate of CD4 cell decline in HIV
	positive men
Passivity/low sense of control	Increased pain and depression in RA patients
	Increased disability and mortality (chronic medical patients)

large volume of literature on stress and illness, race and socioeconomic variables and illness, and the impact of early childhood experiences on adult health.

Stress

Stress is a not only a part of contemporary life but, similar to anxiety, is also intricately connected with our evolution as a species. The theory of natural selection is based on how different species respond to environmental stress. The question of whether stress is bad for our health is a question that many people ponder. Many people have an intuitive sense that stress is bad for them and, especially in urban areas, are drawn to stress-reducing activities such as yoga, meditation, and massage in the hopes of decreasing stress and gaining relaxation. In fact, we are so conditioned to believe that stress is bad for us that patients often tell me that they believe their illnesses were caused by the stress in their lives.

Stress is difficult to study, and there are many different kinds of stress that get studied. Taking care of someone with dementia is one kind of stressor that gets researched; completing a difficult math problem is another. Obviously, there are big differences between stressors, as well as differences in terms of how stressors are evaluated by different people. For example, some people may become very stressed when trying to complete a difficult math problem; others may find the activity fun and challenging. Therefore, the implications of different stressors likely vary from person to person. Further, studies on stress examine both acute and chronic stressors. Although acute stressors do impact the immune system, there is likely to be a difference between the physiological impacts of acute versus chronic stress.

Not only is the topic of stress difficult to study, but it is also hard to know what the research on stress means. Although there are countless studies related to the physiological impact of stress, a frequent criticism of this research is that the markers of stress responses evaluated in studies have questionable clinical significance. As the reader likely knows, humans have been successful as a species because of the flexibility and adaptability of our immune systems. When it fails in one way, it tends to compensate, and especially in young adults, the impact of immune alterations often go unnoticed.

Despite these caveats, it is worth examining some of the findings related to stress, as some of the evidence has potential health implications. Emerging evidence suggests that while stress may not be clinically significant in young people, clinically it can be deleterious as we age or if we develop certain medical illnesses.

There is a relatively long history of studying the effects of stress on the immune system. Research in this area began when it was noticed that certain persons under stress tended to become ill with colds and flu symptoms. A great place to study the physiological impact of stress is in medical schools, as medical schools are filled with healthy young adults who are subjected to both chronic and acute stress. In one study with second year medical students, immune parameters were assessed six weeks prior to exam time and then again during exams. Not only did the researchers find that students were expectedly more emotionally distressed during exam time but they also had lower T and T_H lymphocytes as well as a reduction in NK cells and NK cell cytotoxic activity.[63]

stress. In fact, chronic stress was found to have negative effects of several measures of immune functioning, including neutrophils, eosinophils, monocytes, T-cytotoxic lymphocytes, T-helper cells, as well as the ability to develop antibodies to herpes simplex virus 1. Even though there was a relatively narrow age range in the studies reviewed, it was found that advanced age contributed to altered immune functioning, even during brief stressors. Since normal aging decreases immune functioning, it makes sense that older adults might be more susceptible to stress-related immune functioning. Another review, which looked at stress and the aging immune system, concluded that there is indeed evidence that stress impacts older adults in terms of alterations in different markers of immune functioning.[64]

To my knowledge, one study to date has found that psychological stress increased susceptibility to upper respiratory illness (URI) in otherwise healthy persons.[65] In this creative study by Cohen et al. in 1999, subjects were quarantined for eight days in a hotel and exposed to an infectious dose of an influenza virus. Subjects completed a questionnaire assessing the level of stress that they perceived. Subjects were assessed with both objective markers of illness and subjective experience of symptoms. As the stress in subjects increased, so did symptoms of URI, mucus production, as well as levels of interleukin-6 (IL-6). In HIV patients there is evidence that stress is particularly problematic in terms of disease progression. In a study of HIV-positive men, subjects who were under more stress developed a more rapid course of disease over a period of five years.[66]

Many studies have found that stress impacts the immune system. However, the clinical significance of the stress illness connection remains elusive. It is likely that impact of stress has more severe implications as we age and or when we become ill. Hopefully, the research on stress can begin to focus more on whether the immune changes described above lead to the development of illness in both healthy and medical populations.

Class, Race, and Disparities in Health Care

Despite all of the wonderful advances in medicine in our country and the relative good health of Americans, the unfortunate reality is that health and mortality are often related to factors that people cannot control: their social and economic status and their race. It is very difficult to sort out the impact of race and class because they are often interrelated, but there is much research to support that both of these variables impact health. They probably do so in both similar and different ways. Since entire books have been written on this topic and the history of race and class in the United States is extremely complicated, my aim is to briefly mention some of the issues related to race and class and health care. The reader who would like to get more information regarding the issues should consult the reference list at the end of this chapter.

Class and race inequalities are difficult for most of us to think about. Many people tend to have complicated relationships with money, and in our American culture, consumption, consumerism, and the power of money are tied to our identity in obvious and subtle ways. Additionally, health care professionals, especially physicians, have had to work very hard to get to where they are; the grueling years of training are long and difficult. Although some physicians may come from privileged backgrounds, they still had to suffer through internship and residency like everyone else. In my experience in working with people who have achieved an upper-middle class lifestyle, for some it is hard to think about economic inequalities because they have spent their 20s and 30s getting to a point where they can live comfortably. My point is that we all need money to live, and most of us feel like we do not have enough of it. These issues can make it difficult to think about class differences.

Race is also very difficult for most of us to think about and, of course, is closely tied to class. Perhaps race makes some of us feel more helpless because we have less control over it than we do class. I have noticed when working with professionals who are racial and ethnic minorities, speaking about discrimination is very difficult, not only because it brings up a lot of feelings of anger and sadness but because it creates a sense of helplessness.

Race issues often make us feel guilty if we are Caucasian. Some people keep themselves from feeling guilty by declaring that they do not have any involvement or control over current racial inequality. Additionally, unless

lower classes have greater all-cause mortality rates than people who are in higher classes, and this pattern exists in a stepwise fashion from the poorest to richest.[68] Part of the reason for this may be related to access to affordable and quality health care but this association may also be related to health behaviors. In the United States, persons who do not have a high-school diploma are three times more likely to smoke cigarettes than college graduates.[69] Health behaviors are likely not the whole story, however. Even when factors such as smoking are controlled for, there are still higher rates of mortality in persons earning less money.[70]

Consistent evidence of health care disparities shows that being a member of a racial or ethnic minority is associated with worse outcomes. Although there is a vast amount of research on this topic, it seems that these disparities are due to multiple causes including patient, health care professional, and system attributes.[71] Many studies have been done assessing differences in cardiovascular care. Much of this research has found that African Americans are less likely than whites to receive cardiovascular procedures, and that these differences occur in a variety of settings, including public, private, teaching, and nonteaching hospitals.[72,73] Similar results have been found for Hispanic patients, and Mexican Americans are less likely to receive major medications such as lipid-lowering drugs following an MI.[74,75] The disparities in health care exist across a wide range of medical conditions, from receiving HIV therapies to being placed on transplant waiting lists.[71]

Child Abuse

In addition to race and ethnicity, another factor people cannot control is the family they are raised in. Many health care professionals have probably noticed that some people who come from abusive backgrounds tend to have more difficulties: more psychological problems, more psychosomatic complaints, and perhaps even more "real" physical problems. Research supports these observations, although until recently studies have focused on what we might think of as psychosomatic symptoms. For example, persons who report childhood abuse (usually physical and sexual abuse are surveyed) have more psychosomatic complaints such as chronic pain.[76,77] Additionally, persons with histories of abuse or neglect have more frequent visits to the doctor with medically unexplained symptoms, as compared with individuals without histories of abusive childhood experiences.[78] However, more recent research suggests a link between child abuse and the development of major medical problems. An important study on this topic was published in 1998. Felitti et al., in the Adverse Childhood Experiences Study, surveyed 9,508 adults regarding what they called "adverse childhood experiences."[79] These adverse experiences included child abuse (physical, sexual, or psychological), violence against the respondent's mother, and whether there was someone in the home who was mentally ill, imprisoned, suicidal, or abusing substances. As one might expect, people who had more adverse experiences had increases in psychological problems as well as poor health behaviors. These included alcoholism, drug abuse, depression, suicide attempt, cigarette smoking, poor health, 50-plus sexual partners, and obesity. The second major finding of the study was that there was a "dose response" relationship between the number of adverse events and incidence of ischemic heart disease, cancer, chronic bronchitis or COPD, liver disease, and skeletal fractures.

Another very interesting study on the impact of child abuse and health comes from researchers at Yale University who studied childhood maltreatment and adult cardiovascular disease.[80] These researchers found that a history of childhood abuse or neglect was associated with an almost ninefold increase in cardiovascular disorders in women. Both men and women with histories of abuse or neglect had increases of depression, as might be expected. It was also expected that this history of depression would in part, explain the incidence of heart disease. However, there was no evidence that a history of depression accounted for the prevalence of cardiovascular disease, thus suggesting an independent link between child abuse and cardiovascular disease not explained by depressive symptoms.

Although there are many hypotheses regarding this research, which will be addressed in the next section, part of the explanation is likely the influence of health behaviors. We saw in the Felitti et al. study that persons with multiple adverse childhood experiences were more likely to engage in high-risk health behaviors. Another publication from the Adverse

the development of further illness.

MIND-BODY RELATIONSHIPS: INTEGRATION OF RESEARCH FINDINGS

We have seen a wide range of research that powerfully demonstrates links between emotional states and coping strategies and physical illness. It's hard to fully understand what all of this means, especially because the mechanisms for much of the above research are not well understood. One clue however, comes to us from the child abuse research. People with adverse childhood experiences tend to engage in behaviors that put them at risk for the development of illness. But health behaviors are likely not the whole story. Child abuse is associated with psychopathology such as depression and anxiety disorders such as post-traumatic stress disorder (PTSD). We have seen that certain psychological disorders and emotional states are associated with the development of illness. In the past few years, as these findings have emerged there have been a number of physiological hypotheses developed to try to explain these findings.

One area being studied has to do with cytokines that are released during times of stress, depression, or anxiety. Depression, anxiety, as well as physiological and psychological stress enhance the production of proinflamatory cytokine production, which increases inflammation (This is particularly true for people who are already ill and/or have infections.).[82] Inflammation has been linked with a variety of health problems that are associated with aging, including heart disease, diabetes, hematological malignancies, Alzheimer's disease, arthritis, and osteoporosis.[83] Other aspects of immune functioning in addition to proinflamatory cytokines have been extensively studied. There is evidence of both immune suppression (decreased lymphocytes) and immune activation (increased leukocytes and increased inflammation markers) in major depression.[84]

There has also been an ongoing interest in alterations in endocrine function that occur as a result of emotional responses. Both anxiety and depression result in activation of the hypothalamic–pituitary–adrenal axis (HPA-axis), which causes the release of hormones including the catecholamines, cortisol, prolactin, and growth hormone.[85] These hormones can alter immune functioning, as there is bidirectional feedback between the immune and endocrine systems.[86]

Another area of interest is cardiovascular reactivity. Stress, including marital stress, impacts blood pressure and heart rates, although women appear to be more vulnerable to these effects than men.[87] The effects of chronic cardiovascular arousal are not clearly known; however, it may be that people who are sensitive to increased cardiovascular reactivity may have trouble recovering from that arousal. Once aroused, they may stay that way, leading to other endocrine responses, which may be deleterious for health.

Although much more is unknown than is known regarding the mechanisms of mind–body interactions, research in the last several years has made it more difficult to ignore patient psychological variables that likely play a role in illness development and exacerbation and appear to impact morbidity and mortality. Furthermore, once someone becomes ill, it is clear that coping mechanisms are important. Poor coping, such as passivity and negativity, in addition to lack of social support, is related to less favorable outcomes and symptoms for patients with a variety of illnesses.

All of the mind–body associations that have been discussed may be understood as having complicated bidirectional relationships. We must also keep in mind the powerful role biology plays in the development of any illness. Many people who get depressed or who have had abusive childhoods do not become sick; perhaps those that do have the "right" combination of factors working against them.

Figure 1 is a model of how the mind–body research can be conceptualized. This model represents one hypothesis regarding how physical, psychological, and environmental factors may work together. Since all of the dynamics that contribute to illness are exceedingly complex, this model is an attempt to synthesize all of the research that has been presented and is not meant to suggest direct cause and effect relationships.

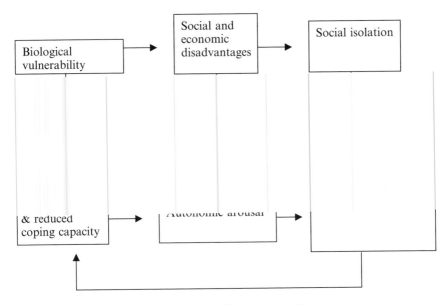

Figure 1. Possible mechanisms of mind-body associations.

Biological vulnerability, in combination with early childhood adversity do make people vulnerable to both specific psychopathologies such as depression, but probably also to autonomic arousal, and both may create a physiological environment in which illness can develop. Poor coping and health behaviors may increase this vulnerability. Social isolation may cause more physiological arousal, thus creating risk for illness, but from a practical standpoint, people who are alone do not get encouragement to take care of themselves such as making doctor appointments, remembering to take medication, etc. Additionally, persons who do not have access to health care and those who are economically disadvantaged may be at higher risk for not taking care of themselves and may also be isolated due to feeling marginalized by society. Once someone becomes ill, the impact of poor coping, poor health behaviors, and psychopathology may be more detrimental. Additionally, getting sick is stressful and can lead to depression and anxiety. Illness also reduces access to social support and creates isolation.

The relationships between the factors described are complex and it is likely that feedback loops exist between them. Figure 1 places a fair of amount consideration on early childhood experiences. This is due in part to known prevalence of child abuse, which increases illness vulnerability but also to emerging neurological research, which demonstrates that neurological development is impacted greatly by children's attachments to their caregivers.[88] Much of this research suggests that patterns of arousal and coping are developed in response to early environmental factors. I suspect that many people who have not been abused develop a tendency toward increased autonomic arousal and/or depression and anxiety. Relationships are extremely complicated, and, as we all know, stress in response to relationships happens often not in the context of what we would think of as abuse. It seems to be part of the human condition that we do not always get along with the people we love. Additionally, children are born with different temperaments, and not all children and caretakers fit well with each other. For these reasons, I suspect that particular kinds of stresses in childhood make people vulnerable to illness and that abuse is only one of these stresses.

CONCLUSIONS

A large body of research powerfully links psychological and physical functioning, although the mechanisms regarding these associations are unclear. Some of the most replicated research relates to depression. Depression is linked with heart disease and mortality in older adults. It is unknown if depression is causal in these associations or if depression signs and symptoms are expressions of underlying disease processes. Interestingly, at the time of this writing, I have not seen research that demonstrates that treating major depression with medication or psychotherapy improves mortality outcomes in heart disease patients. We have also seen that hostility and cynicism impact health, especially in terms of atherosclerotic disease. Although anxiety is much more difficult to study, certain types of anxiety are associated with sudden cardiac death and heart disease.

Persons who can utilize social support, have satisfying relationships, maintain a positive attitude, and find meaning or even benefit from their illness tend to have better psychological and physical outcomes. Certain stresses early in life combined with biological vulnerability increase physiological arousal as well as the tendency to engage in negative health behaviors, which could increase physiological vulnerability to illness.

This kind of research can tempt us to make simple cause and effect relationships between emotional factors and illness, but my work with young adults who develop hematological malignancies has taught me about the random cruelty of illness. Although this research can help us to understand how psychological factors may contribute to or exacerbate illness, we are far from explanations regarding what causes many of the illnesses that harm us.

organized emotional and coping topics, in reality it is difficult to separate some of these constructs. For example, feeling "stressed" and feeling anxious may have a number of similarities, and anxiety may manifest itself differently among individuals. Further, some persons with depression may experience physiological arousal secondary to anxious rumination, while others may be profoundly anergic and have hypersomnia and may not have physiological arousal at all. Therefore, there are limits to our attempts to define and organize psychological constructs in this way, as well as limits to how we might interpret the research findings. Finally, it is likely that there are factors that influence health that have not been thoroughly studied. For example, sleep disturbance is a common denominator for some people who are stressed, anxious, or depressed, and perhaps we will find that sleep disturbance has negative immunologic and/or cardiovascular effects.

One of the main conclusions we can draw from this research is that the mind influences the body and vice versa. For our work with patients, this research can remind us to consider psychological factors when working with people who are healthy or ill. This research may also justify more aggressive treatment of mood disorders, as doing so could theoretically impact later physical health.

REFERENCES

1. American Psychological Association. Summit on women and depression Presented at Wye River conference center; 2002.
2. Sartorius N, Üstün TB, Lecrubier Y, et al. Depression co-morbid with anxiety: results from the WHO study on psychological disorders in primary health care. *Br J Psychiatry.* 1996;168(suppl 30):38–43.

3. Frasure-Smith N, Lesperance F, Talajic M. Depression following myocardial infarction: impact on 6-month survival. *JAMA*. 1993;270:1819–1824.

4. Barefoot JC, Brummett BH, Helms MJ, et al. Depressive symptoms and survival of patients with coronary artery disease. *Psychosom Med*. 2000;62:790–795.

5. Jiang W, Alexander J, Christopher E, et al. Relationship of depression to increased risk of mortality and rehospitalization in patients with congestive heart failure. *Arch Intern Med*. 2001;161:1849–1856.

6. Ford DE, Mead LA, Chang PP, et al. Depression is a risk factor for coronary artery disease in men: the John Hopkins precursors study. *Arch Intern Med*. 1998;158:1422–1426.

7. Glassman AH, Shapiro PA. Depression and the course of coronary artery disease. *Am J Psychiatry*. 1998;155:4–11.

8. Pratt LA, Ford DE, Crum RM, et al. Depression, psychotropic medication and risk of myocardial infarction. *Circulation*. 1996;94:3123–3129.

9. Bush DE, Ziegelstein RC, Tayback M, et al. Even minimal symptoms of depression increase mortality risk after acute myocardial infarction. *Am J Cardiol*. 2001;88:337–341.

10. Penninx BWJH, Guralnik JM, Ferucci L, et al. Depressive symptoms and physical decline in community dwelling older persons. *JAMA*. 1998;279:1720–1726.

11. Herrmann C, Brand-Driehorst S, Kaminsky B, et al. Diagnostic groups and depressed mood as predictors of 22-month mortality in medical inpatients. *Psychosom Med*. 1998;60:570–577.

12. Whooley MA, Browner WS. Association between depressive symptoms and mortality in older women. *Arch Intern Med*. 1998;158:2129–2135.

13. McGee R, Williams S, Elwood M. Depression and the development of cancer: a meta-analysis. *Soc Sci Med*. 1994;38:187–192.

14. Penninx BWJH, Guralnik JM, Pahor M, et al. Chronically depressed mood and cancer risk in older persons. *J Natl Cancer Inst*. 1998;90:1888–1893.

15. Giese-Davis J, Spiegel D. Emotional expression and cancer progression. In: Davidson RJ, Scherer K, Hill H, et al., eds. *Handbook of Affective Sciences*. Oxford: Oxford University Press; 2003:1053–1082.

16. Montazeri A, Jarvandi S, Ebrahimi M, et al. The role of depression in the development of breast cancer: analysis of registry data from a single institute. *Asian Pac J Cancer Prev*. 2004;5:316–319.

17. Gallo JJ, Armenian HK, Ford DE, et al. Major depression and cancer: the 13-year follow-up of the Baltimore epidemiologic catchment area sample. *Cancer Causes Control*. 2000;11:751–758.

18. Spiegel D, Giese-Davis J. Depression and cancer: mechanisms and disease progression. *Biol Psychiatry*. 2003;54:269–282.

19. Jacka FN, Pasco JA, Henry MJ, et al. Depression and bone mineral density in a community sample of perimenopausal women: Geelong osteoporosis study. *Menopause*. 2005;12:88–91.

20. Kahl KG, Rudolf S, Stoeckelhuber BM, et al. Bone mineral density markers of bone turnover, and cytokines in young women with borderline personality disorder with and without comorbid major depressive disorder. *Am J Psychiatry.* 2005;162:168–174.

logic follow-up study. *Public Health Rep.* 2005;120:71–75.

24. Kubzansky LD, Kawachi I, Weiss ST, et al. Anxiety and coronary heart disease: a synthesis of epidemiological, psychological, and experimental evidence. *Ann Behav Med.* 1998;20:47–58.

25. Huffman JC, Pollack MH, Stern TA. Panic disorder and chest pain: mechanisms morbidity and management. Primary Care Companion *J Clin Psychiatry.* 2002;4:54–62.

26. Suls J, Bunde J. Anger, anxiety, and depression as risk factors for cardiovascular disease: the problems and implications of overlapping affective dispositions. *Psychol Bull.* 2005;131:260–300.

27. Kawachi I, Colditz GA, Acherio A, et al. Prospective study of phobic anxiety and CHD in men. *Circulation.* 1994;89:1992–1997.

28. Albert C, Chae CU, Rexrode KM, et al. Phobic anxiety and risk of coronary heart disease and sudden cardiac death among women. *Circulation.* 2005;111:480–487.

29. Friedman M, Rosenman RH. *Type A Behavior and Your Heart.* New York: Knopf; 1974.

30. Cook W, Medley D. Proposed hostility and pharisaic virtue scales for the MMPI. *J Appl Psychol.* 1954;238:414–418.

31. Rozanski A, Blumenthal JA, Kaplan J. Impact of psychological factors on the pathogenesis of cardiovascular disease and implications for therapy. *Circulation.* 1999;99:2192–2217.

32. Myrtek M. Meta-analysis of prospective studies on coronary heart disease, type A personality and hostility. *Int J Cardiol.* 2001;79:245–251.

33. Smith TW, Glazer K, Ruiz JM, et al. Hostility, anger, aggressiveness, and coronary heart disease: an interpersonal perspective on personality, emotion, and health. *J Pers.* 2004;72:1217–1270.

34. Moller J, Hallqvist J, Diderichsen F, et al. Do episodes of anger trigger myocardial infarction? A case crossover analysis in the Stockholm heart epidemiology program (SHEEP). *Psychosom Med.* 1999;61:842–849.

35. Lepore SJ. Cynicism, social support, and cardiovascular reactivity. *Health Psychol.* 1995;14:210–216.

36. Benotsch EG, Christensen AJ, McKelvey L. Hostility, social support, and ambulatory cardiovascular activity. *J Behav Med.* 1997;20:163–182.

37. Iribarren C, Sidney S, Bild D, et al. Association of hostility with coronary artery calcification in young adults. *JAMA.* 2000;283:2546–2551.

38. Rees WD, Lutkins SG. Mortality of bereavement. *Br Med J.* 1967;4:13–16.

39. Case RB, Moss AJ, Case N, et al. Living alone after myocardial infarction. *JAMA.* 1992;267:515–519.

40. Ruberman W, Weinblatt E, Goldberg JD, et al. Psychosocial influences on mortality after myocardial infarction. *N Engl J Med.* 1984;311:552–559.

41. Mookadam F, Arthur HM. Social support and its relationship to morbidity and mortality after acute myocardial infarction. *Arch Intern Med.* 2004;164:1514–1518.

42. Hous JS, Landis KR, Umberson D. Social relationships and health. *Science.* 1988;241:540–545.

43. Berkman LF. Social networks, host resistance and mortality: a 9-year follow-up of Alameda County residents. *Am J Epidemiol.* 1979;109:186–204.

44. Pressman SD, Cohen S, Miller GE, et al. Loneliness, social network size, and immune response to influenza vaccine in college freshman. *Health Psychol.* 2005;24:297–306.

45. Kiecolt-Glaser JK, Newton TL. Marriage and health: his and hers. *Psychol Bull.* 2001;127:472–503.

46. Smith TB, McCullough ME, Poll J. Religiousness and depression: evidence for a main effect and the moderating influence of life events. *Psychol Bull.* 2003;129:614–636.

47. Burker EJ, Evon DM, Sedway JA, et al. Religious coping, psychological distress and disability among patients with end stage pulmonary disease. *J Clin Psychol Med Setttings.* 2004;11:179–193.

48. Hughes JW, Tomilnson A, Blumenthal JA, et al. Social support and religiousity as coping strategies for anxiety in hospitalized cardiac patients. *Ann Behav Med.* 2004;28:179–185.

49. Pargament KI. *The Psychology of Religion and Coping: Theory, Research and Practice.* New York: Guilford; 1997.

50. Harrison M, Koenig HG, Hays J, et al. The epidemiology of religious coping: a review of recent literature. *Int Rev Psychiatry.* 2001;13:86–93.

51. Bolger N, Eckenrode J. Social relationships, personality, and anxiety during a major stressful event. *J Pers Soc Psychol.* 1991;61:440–449.

52. Marsland AL, Cohen S, Rabin BS, et al. Associations between stress, trait negative affect, and acute immune reactivity and antibody response to hepatitis B injection in healthy young adults. *Health Psychol.* 2001;20:4–11.

53. Reed GM, Kemeny ME, Taylor SE, et al. Negative HIV specific expectancies and AIDS related bereavement as predictors of symptom onset an asymptomatic HIV positive gay men. *Health Psychol.* 1999;18:354–363.

54. Kamen-Siegel L, Rodin J, Seligman MEP, et al. Explanatory style and cell medi-

2005;10:457–474.

58. Carver CS, Antoni MH. Finding benefit in breast cancer during the first year after diagnosis predicts better adjustment 5–8 years after diagnosis. *Health Psychol.* 2004;23:595–598.

59. Bower JE, Kemeny ME, Taylor SE, et al. Cognitive processing discovery of meaning, CD4 decline and AIDS related mortality among bereaved HIV seropositive men. *J Consult Clin Psychol.* 1998;66:979–986.

60. Covic J, Adamson B, Hough M. The impact of passive coping on rheumatoid arthritis pain. *Rheumatology.* 2000;39:1027–1030.

61. Nusselder WJ, Looman CWN, Mackenbach JP. Nondisease factors affected trajectories of disability in a prospective study. *J Clin Epidemiol.* 2005;58:484–494.

62. Glaser R, Kiecolt-Glaser JK, Stout JC, et al. Stress related impairments in cellular immunity. *Psychiatry Res.* 1985;16:233–239.

63. Segerstrom SC, Miller GE. Psychological stress and the human immune system: a meta analytic study of 30 years of inquiry. *Psychol Bull.* 2004;130:601–630.

64. Hawkley LC, Cacioppo JT. Stress and the aging immune system. *Brain Behav Immun.* 2004;18:114–119.

65. Cohen S, Doyle WJ, Skoner DP. Psychological stress cytokine production and severity of upper respiratory illness. *Psychsom Med.* 1999;61:175–180.

66. Lesserman J, Jackson ED, Peitto JM, et al. Progression to AIDS: the effects of stress, depressive symptoms, and social support. *Psychosom Med.* 1999;61:397–406.

67. Starfield B. Is United States health really the best in the world? *JAMA.* 2000; 284:483–485.

68. McDonough P, Duncan GJ, Williams DR, et al. Income dynamics and adult mortality in the United States, 1972–1989. *Am J Pub Health.* 1997;87:1476–1483.

69. Health: United States, Hyattsville, MD. *National Center for Health Statistics.* 198 DHHS publication, 2002-1232; 2002.

70. Davey-Smith G, Blane D, Bartly M. Explanations for socioeconomic differentials in mortality: evidence from Britain and elsewhere. *Eur J Pub Health.* 1994;94:131–144.

71. Institute of Medicine of the National Academies. *Unequal Treatment: Confronting Racial and Ethnic Disparities in Health care.* Washington, DC: The National Academies Press; 2003.

72. Ford ES, Cooper R, Castaner A, et al. Cornorary arteriography and cornonary bypass among whites and other racial groups relative to hospital-based-incidence rates for coronary artery disease: finding from NHDS. *Am J Pub Health.* 1998;79:437–440.

73. Ayanian JZ, Udvarhelyi IS, Gatsonis CA, et al. Racial differences in the use of revascularization procedures after coronary angiography. *JAMA.* 1993;269:2642–2646.

74. Carlisle DM, Leake BD, Shapiro MF. Racial and ethnic differences in the use of invasive cardiac procedures among cardiac patients in Los Angeles County, 1986 through 1988. *Am J Pub Health.* 1995;85:352–356.

75. Herholz H, Goff DC, Ramsey DJ, et al. Women and Mexican Americans receive fewer cardiovascular drugs following myocardial infarction than men and non-Hispanic whites: the Corpus Christi heart project, 1988–1990. *J Clin Epidemol.* 1996;49:279–287.

76. Wurtele SK, Kaplan GM, Keairnes M. Childhood sexual abuse among chronic pain patients. *Clin J Pain.* 1990;6:110–113.

77. Walker EA, Katon WJ, Harrop-Griffithss J, et al. Relationship of chronic pelvic pain to psychiatric diagnoses and childhood sexual abuse. *Am J Psychiatry.* 1998;145:75–80.

78. Fiddler M, Phil M, Jackson J, et al. Childhood adversity and frequent medical consultations. *Gen Hosp Psychiatry.* 2004;26:367–377.

79. Felitti VJ, Anda RF, Nordenberg D, et al. Relationship of childhood abuse and household dysfunction to many leading causes of death in adults. *Am J Prev Med.* 1998;14:245–258.

80. Balben SV, Aslan M, Maciejewski PK. Childhood maltreatment as a risk factor for adult cardiovascular disease and depression. *J Clin Psychiatry.* 2004;65:249–254.

81. Dube SR, Felitti VJ, Dong M, et al. The impact of adverse childhood experiences on health problems: evidence from birth cohorts dating back to 1900. *Prev Med.* 2003;37:268–277.

82. Kiecolt-Glaser JK, McGuire L, Robles TF, et al. Emotions morbidity and mortality: new perspectives from psychoneuroimmunology. *Annu Rev Psychol.* 2002;53:83–107.

83. Ershler W, Keller E. Age associated increased interleukin-6 gene expression, late life diseases and frailty. *Annu Rev Med.* 2000;51:245–270.

84. Raison CL, Miller AH. The neuroimmunology of stress and depression. *Sem Clin Neuropsychiatry.* 2001;6:277–294.

85. Miller AH. Neuroendocrine and immune system interactions in stress and depression. *Psychiatr Clin North Am.* 1998;21:443–463.

86. Rabin BS. *Stress Immune Function and Health: the Connection.* New York: Wiley, 1999.

87. Robles TF, Kiecolt-Glaser J. The physiology of marriage: pathways to health. *Phyisol Behav.* 2003;79:409–416.

2

DOCTORS AND PAT...

"*The irony is that the healthier Western society becomes, the more medicine it craves.*"

—Roy Porter

While the previous chapter described some of the major research linking mental states and physical functioning and provided an empirical rationale for the need to address patient's psychological and emotional issues, actually addressing emotional issues in medical settings is difficult. Consider the following case example:

> Susan is a 52-year-old Caucasian female who has seen her primary care physician for the last 4 years. Current medical problems include hypertension, osteoarthritis, and chronic low back pain. She is 60 pounds overweight, and although her doctor has told her that her medical problems would improve if she lost weight, she has not. In fact, she has gained 5 pounds since her last visit. She presents for the current visit because she has had frequent urination and excessive thirst and hunger. Her blood analysis shows hyperglycemia (glucose = 234) as well as an increase in her low-density lipoprotein (LDL = 180). Her diagnosis is Type II diabetes. When discussing these lab findings, Susan reports to her physician that she has been very stressed at work. She works at a

desk job in middle management and is having trouble with her employees and her boss. As her doctor tries to talk with her about necessary dietary changes she will need to make, she bursts out crying and says, "I can't change my eating habits, I have tried and nothing works!" Further inquiry reveals that she is currently getting divorced after finding out that her husband has had an affair. Additionally, her 23-year-old son who lives with her has just been arrested for driving drunk. Her physician, Dr. Smith, feels sympathetic, yet overwhelmed and slightly irritated by Susan's emotional outburst. With a waiting room full of patients, she suggests to Susan that a therapist might be able to help her with her problems. Susan stops crying and says she will think about seeing a mental health professional. Dr. Smith continues on with directions regarding dietary and activity changes.

Some of the obstacles to addressing emotional issues in medical practice are simply related to time and the need to prioritize issues addressed based on acuity. For example, Susan has acute medical issues that need to be discussed. While her social situation is highly problematic, addressing these issues in depth during the above meeting would not allow time for her physician to address the more immediate concern of hyperglycemia. Other barriers to addressing emotional issues in patients are far subtler and are based on how we think about the origin of physical problems and psychological problems. This chapter will address the context in which practicing medicine takes place, the complicated aspects of the culture of medicine, and physician and patient satisfaction. I will also discuss the impact of technology on the practice of medicine, resulting in a number of changes in how physicians of today's generation practice. Although I will be largely describing aspects of medical practice in the United States, much of what I describe is applicable to all countries that utilize Western medical principles.

SCIENCE AND THE CULTURE OF MEDICINE

While many would argue that the practice of medicine is an art, Western medicine is deeply rooted in the scientific tradition. Although this fact is so obvious that it barely warrants articulation, science is a particular philosophy that influences the way we think and is the guiding principle in the medical treatment of patients. Since we all learn scientific principles in medical school and graduate school, we take the assumptions of science so much for granted that we often do not stop to think about the meaning of

4. Causes of disease are biological and do not result as a product of consciousness or mental states.

Appling these principles to Susan, we know what is physically wrong with her based on our observations (we can see she is obese) and her lab tests (high LDL, elevated glucose). We can predict that based on her current health status she is at risk for the development of heart disease. Her excessive thirst and hunger and her frequent urination are all attributable to her Type-II diabetes. Finally, many physicians would not implicate her stressful and chaotic social situation in her development of diabetes.

Western medicine as we know it today has its roots in ancient Greece. Hippocrates and others developed a model of health and illness in terms of humors, and illness was determined by whether these fluids remained in balance. Galen, who lived a few hundred years later (AD 129 to circa 216), was both a philosopher and physician and espoused medicine as the involvement of empirical science, ethics, and philosophical discourse.[1] The importance of human anatomy was expanded by Leonardo da Vinci, Marcantonio, and Vesalius through human dissections; these observations could confirm or refute what had been previously speculated regarding anatomy and physiology.[2] Much of how we think about the science of Western medicine, however, is attributed to René Descartes, who lived from 1596 to 1650. He stated that the mind and the body are subject to different laws of causality based on his proposition that the body exists in space and the mind exists in time.[3] Descartes' theory became known as *dualism*, and his writing on this topic is a bit confusing. While Descartes did suggest that causal interactions between the mind and body take place, they are subject to different laws of causality. The latter part of this apparent contradiction has resulted in the main interpretation of

Descartes' position on the "mind–body problem." A dualistic stance is usually interpreted to mean that the mind and the body are separate and do not influence one another. Dualism fits well with scientific principles because anatomy, bodily processes, cell growth, and regeneration can all be readily observed. The development of science in the Western world, as well as the embracing of technology by the United States, has led to the creation of the current medical system.

How does the philosophy of Western medicine pertain to our present discussion of the context of medical practice in the United States? The philosophical underpinnings of medicine are likely responsible for the "compartmentalization" that exists in medicine today. Offices for physical doctors and offices for mental health doctors are often in separate buildings, reflecting the dualistic idea that the mind and the body operate in separate realms. In medical practice, some physicians rarely have contact with psychiatrist colleagues; psychiatry still tends to be a less desirable specialty among medical students choosing residencies. Psychiatrists also tend to remark that they feel less valued than other physicians that they are at the bottom of the physician hierarchy.

The way we separate the mind and the body is also mirrored in medical research, which strives to understand the infinitely complex nature of the human body. One example of this relates to the understanding of the immune system. Because immune cells possess a unique ability to grow outside of the human body, it was concluded that the immune system functions separately from the other systems in the body.[4] We now understand, however, that the immune system is greatly influenced by other systems in the body, especially the endocrine system. As described in Chapter 1, these interactions are thought to partially explain the connection between emotions and illness.

Compartmentalization is also evident in the specialization of medicine. Since our understanding of disease processes has expanded exponentially in the last few decades, physicians have become highly specialized. While this specialization has obvious benefits, it can be limiting in that patients often have multiple providers who each focus on one specific part of the body. For patients with multiple medical problems, this can create a situation in which there are multiple providers who may have different ideas about the origin of illness or even what treatment methods should be undertaken. Although in the majority of cases clinicians work collaboratively to bridge the separation of specialized fields, sometimes communication falters and patients feel confused about who is directing their treatment.

The split between academic medicine and clinical medicine also reflects the separation of two compartmentalized fields. The

example, research studies often use instruments not familiar to clinicians and ask research questions that do not seem relevant to the day-to-day issues of practice. While both medical and psychological research may be interesting, clinicians in general want information that is readily accessible, is relevant to patient care, and that uses familiar language.

The tendency to cognitively separate information into smaller units is a common coping strategy. In our age of overwhelming information stimulation, compartmentalizing keeps us from getting overwhelmed. In terms of how we think about physical and psychological functioning, breaking information down makes it easier to come up with conclusions. For example, if I have a headache, I might try to determine if the cause has psychological or physical roots. If I decide that my headache is stress related, my diagnosis is a tension headache; I will try to relax. On the other hand, if I have the worst headache of my life, I may suspect an impending aneurism and rush to the emergency room. Once I decide whether the cause is physical or psychological, I have a better sense of how to behave. The way we naturally separate the mind and the body is an efficient form of cognitive processing that makes it easier for us to understand the world as well as our bodies. When something has both physical and psychological influences, it is much more difficult to think about and it makes it hard to know what behaviors to undertake to solve the problem. Let us return to Susan. If her doctor thinks of her health problems as purely biological, the treatment plan is relatively straightforward; she needs to make dietary changes, or she will likely need insulin. Her doctor needs to encourage her to change her diet as well as increase her activity level and counsel her on the consequences of not doing so. The fact that Susan needs to make major behavioral adjustments (not just taking medication) makes her situation more difficult. The fact that she is unlikely to make any of these changes makes her situation much more frustrating. Add a diagnosis of depression to the picture, and now her physician has to come up with a plan for treating the depression. In thinking about the origin of her illnesses, considering depression as well as the impact of her chronic stress makes her case more complicated. And many physicians might ask how does thinking about the relationship of depression and her illnesses affect the treatment plan? How will it change the outcome? It is difficult for physicians to deal with patients who have preventable medical problems. Addressing psychological needs can add to a sense of futility. With patients who have trouble making behavioral changes or who have emotional contributions to their illnesses, physicians can feel frustrated at addressing problems that may never be resolved. One woman, a real-life Susan, recently told me, while sobbing, that three of her doctors had told her that she will die within 5 years if she didn't lose weight and change her activity level. Such situations are frustrating for both doctors and patients who very much want change but don't know how to make it happen. These types of situations with patients make it very difficult to think of the impact of emotions because there is so much else to try to manage.

WORKING IN MEDICINE TODAY: A CRISIS IN HEALTH CARE?

Practicing medicine today involves a number of unique stresses. These stresses involve changes in the political, economic, technological, and social aspects of being a doctor.

The experience of practicing medicine now is very different than it was for physicians of preceding generations. Abigail Zuger provided a concise summary of changes in medicine in a *New England Journal of Medicine* article on physician dissatisfaction:[5]

> The profession of medicine has taken its members on a wild ride during the past century: a slow glorious climb in well being followed by a steep stomach-churning fall. In the decades after World War II, sociologists portrayed American doctors as the lucky heirs to a golden age of medicine. They were surrounded by admiring assistants, loyal patients, and respectful colleagues and had full autonomy in their work, job security, and a luxurious income.

This era was short-lived. By the 1980s, newspaper headlines proclaimed that many of the nations "dispirited doctors" were considering bailing out of medicine, and subsequent observers have continued to describe a profession in retreat, plagued by bureaucracy, loss of autonomy

the context in which medicine is practiced. Although the changes in medicine are multifaceted, many surveys of physicians implicate managed care as a source of discontent. In contrast to previous generations, physicians today are faced with the pressures of cost containment in addition to providing patient care. The pressures of managed care are associated with physician dissatisfaction through a loss of autonomy, difficulties in maintaining an ethical practice, "gate keeping" (in primary care), an increased sense of competition, as well as difficulty in establishing patient trust.[6,7]

Related to the influence of managed care, the financial culture of medicine has changed in the last several years. Many physicians feel pressured to see more patients in order to earn a living. While it is unclear if reimbursements have decreased across all fields of medicine, or whether reimbursement has not increased with the cost of living, some physicians do not feel appropriately compensated for their work. A survey of family practice doctors found that almost one-third of respondents did not feel satisfied with compensation.[8] Perhaps due to the influence of managed care or the need for more aggressive marketing, physicians are required to do more work now (administrative tasks) than before, thus requiring more work that is not compensated. Even if financial reimbursement has been stable, the increasingly high cost of living in many urban areas and the burden of medical school loans exacerbate financial worries.

Another major change in medicine in the United States is the high cost of medical care. This is sometimes attributed to physicians' over-utilization of diagnostic tests and procedures.[9] While it may be true that reducing clinical interventions could help with health care costs, it is important to remember that changes in patient expectations may be related to health care costs. As people live longer and as Americans become more affluent, the tendency of patients to focus on health is likely to increase. Presently, pressure on physicians to act in response to patient anxieties about bodily concerns is enormous. Additionally, the tendency among many physicians is to be thorough and to make sure all possibilities of illness are ruled out, thus increasing the likelihood of unnecessary diagnostic tests or procedures. The rising incidence of medical malpractice probably reinforces this tendency. It is also the case that medical practice in the United States is based on a very proactive model. One physician author described the situation as: "The dominant response to a presenting illness [in the United States] is to do something ('don't just stand there, do something')".[9]

My own experience in hospitals has reflected this. I notice that when I am in the hospital, I walk fast, talk fast, and think fast. I feel pressure to do everything in a hurry, although there is often no rational reason for me to feel this way. There is a very real sense of time urgency in many hospitals, and I suspect that this reflects the attitude of "doing something." Working with medical patients is difficult in a number of ways. Perhaps continually moving, both intellectually and physically, makes the work of caring for patients more manageable.

TECHNOLOGY, RELATIONSHIPS, AND PHYSICIAN AUTHORITY

Another major shift in medicine is the impact of technology on how medicine is practiced. The field of medicine has always been an inspiration for curious people. Medical students talk with amazement about the intricacies of the body, as well as the body's capacity for healing itself. The field of medicine now involves much more than learning disease signs and symptoms. Medicine has expanded exponentially in the use of technology and, with this, the ability to eradicate illness and/or prolong life. Technology is now such a part of how medicine is practiced that it is impossible to imagine medicine before MRI scanning, CT scanning, transplant surgeries, in vitro fertilization, and angioplasty. Technology has many implications. First, it affords more options for physicians to diagnose and treat disease. More than ever before, physicians have new tools for diagnosing diseases that would have been missed (using PET scans to detect early cancer relapse is one example). Technology also creates ethical dilemmas. Examples include the supply and demand for solid organs and the ability to keep persons in the intensive care unit alive with ventilators, pressors, and antibiotics. Another challenge associated with technology is that it may have changed the pressure placed on physicians. The technological miracles in our affluent country provide the illusion that technology can

Because technology can increase expectations placed on physicians and is a major part of the practice of medicine today, it also changes the doctor–patient relationship. Physicians are drawn to medicine in part because they value human relationships; they care about patients and want to heal. The doctor–patient relationship is an essential part of the work for most health care clinicians. For any of us who work with patients, relationships are integral to day-to-day satisfaction. A difficult patient can cause us to have a bad afternoon, while a patient who makes positive changes due to our influence is a major source of satisfaction and esteem. Although technology and the basics of caring for patients can be complementary, they can also be in conflict, and this impacts the doctor–patient relationship. While technology heals and allows physicians to practice in an historically unprecedented way, it creates an environment in which procedures and advanced diagnostic equipment have a role in the provision of patient care. Many diagnostic and treatment procedures are physically intrusive and uncomfortable for patients. For most physicians, some emotional detachment is required in order to continue to do procedures everyday. For example, cardiac catheterization is quite uncomfortable for patients, even with conscious sedation. Doctors who perform these procedures need to concentrate and keep the patient from moving so they can identify culprit arterial lesions. Some level of detachment is necessary for the physician to be able to focus on the procedure. In addition, a doctor who focuses too much on patient discomfort may have difficulty performing uncomfortable procedures. Performing cardiac catheterization is very different than conducting a routine follow-up visit for hypertension, when the doctor can be more available for some emotional connection with the patient. The technological aspects of medicine change relationships with patients as physicians have varying roles to play that are different than early twentieth century doctors who made house calls. In the past, the provision of emotional support was primary. One probable consequence of technology is that it is less frequently possible for physicians to provide emotional support to patients. Often this is not congruent with the importance of relationships, which matter to both doctors and patients.

Another difficulty with practicing medicine today is that while physicians are idealized and expected to perform miracles, as the letter to the *British Medical Journal* illustrates, medicine and doctors are simultaneously devalued. Though doctors once had the ultimate authority to determine diagnostic tests and treatments, many physicians have their recommendations reviewed by insurance companies to determine medical necessity. Additionally, hospital administrators pressure medical staff to reduce the length of hospital stays. This is not unlike what has happened in the field of psychology and psychiatry. Insurance companies frequently interrupt treatments because they determine that the number of sessions exceeds medical necessity. Many therapists and psychiatrists choose not to accept insurance for this reason and see only cash-paying patients. This is rarely an option for medical doctors; the high cost of medical care prohibits abandoning insurance.

Having treatment plans reviewed is one way practicing medicine is less satisfying. The rise in reports of medical errors is another. Newspaper articles have been reporting on medical errors for a number of years and call into question physician authority. While medical errors are serious and should be treated as such, a consequence of these stories is that patients increasingly mistrust their doctor.

A number of conflicts are associated with being a physician today. Physicians are both idealized and devalued. The aspect of patient care that involves the relationship between the patient and the doctor is very difficult to maintain due to changes in the culture of medicine. Managed care is one of these changes and creates a scenario in which physicians' individual autonomy and decision-making ability is reduced. Technology feeds the illusion of abolishing mortality and creates unrealistic expectations of physician abilities. The use of technology also places doctors in multiple roles and requires flexibility in emotional availability or detachment. In some ways, due to the advances in medical care, doctors are more valuable than ever. On the other hand, the stakes are higher now. The promise of medicine creates higher expectations than at any other

limited our bodies are. Acknowledging the inherent limitations of our bodies is very difficult for all but excruciating and humiliating for some. These dynamics will be described in later chapters related to individual psychology, but the illusion of modern medicine giving us unlimited bodily potential is quite seductive.

Perhaps the cultural changes described above are associated with patient dissatisfaction with medical care in the United States. More patients than ever before are turning outside of the medical system and utilizing alternative medicine. The use of alternative medicine increased dramatically in the 1990s. From 1990 to 1997, alternative medicine use increased from 36.3 percent to 46.3 percent.[11] The reasons for this are complicated but likely involve a number of factors including increases in chronic diseases, reduction in respect for authoritarian professions, increased access to health information, and desire for a better quality of life.[12] There is also evidence that dissatisfaction with Western medicine is associated with patient use of alternative medicine, although this has not been demonstrated consistently.[13–15]

While there has always been a subgroup of people in the United States who have utilized alternative medicine approaches, the sharp rise in alternative approaches including the use of herbal remedies suggests a desire among patients to take control of medical problems. While in some ways this increase in patient control can be construed as a healthy form of patient empowerment, it suggests a departure from the previous views of physicians as all-knowing and wise. Authority is a crucial aspect of many professional relationships. We need to feel confident in the abilities of those we ask to help us. However, changes in access to health information have changed perceptions of physician authority. People now routinely turn to the Internet to inquire about physical signs and symptoms.

Many of these people feel that they have a good idea of what is wrong with them before even seeing their doctor for a consultation. Access to the Internet and health information reduces the power differential between doctors and patients. Doctors' recommendations can be checked easily, and patients with similar diseases can communicate over e-mail and in chat rooms regarding how their treatments might differ. Patients then ask doctors about their care. This kind of inquiry is relatively new to health care and can be frustrating for physicians. Patients might ask why they are not receiving a certain treatment when that treatment isn't indicated for the specific problem. In this way, the ideas that most of us have grown up with, that physicians have ultimate authority, have begun to erode.

The issue of patient satisfaction has many facets. Being unhappy with medical treatment is much different than being unhappy with a relationship with a doctor. As a psychologist who sees many medical patients, I have heard a number of patients complain about their doctors. (In most cases, patients do not say anything to their doctors about their concerns. This is especially true among surgery patients and persons who are seriously ill.) The majority of complaints that I hear have nothing to do with medical treatment decisions but are focused on the quality of the interpersonal relationship with the doctor. For example, patients often complain that their doctors do not spend enough time with them. I have heard this complaint regarding both inpatient and outpatient contacts. When doctors do spend a lot of time with patients, patients speak of this very highly. They appear to be happy with the idea that their doctor "cares enough" to spend time with them. In an empirical study of patient perceptions of time with their primary care doctors in the United Kingdom, half of the study patients (150 people) wanted more time with their doctors, but many of these patients tended to underestimate the amount of time they actually spent with their physician.[16] The results of this study found that the desire for more time with a physician was not associated with satisfaction with the visit, physician information giving, or the physical examination. The study participants who wanted more time with their doctors were not satisfied with the emotional content of the visit, suggesting that it is an emotional connection that patients crave with their doctors and that it is the quality of interactions, not the length of the visit, that is fundamentally important to patients. Indeed, other studies have not found that physicians are spending less time with patients.[17]

Despite changes in patient perceptions of medicine, people still very much need their doctors to treat them. Although some people become overly dependent on their doctors (this will be discussed in subsequent chapters) the reality is that physicians...

...however, takes its toll. Accounts of physicians who make medical mistakes and then think frequently about them years later are one illustration of this. Strife in physician marriages is another.[18]

ADDRESSING EMOTIONS IN THE CONTEXT OF MODERN MEDICINE

Being a health care provider today is as exciting as it is frustrating. The pressures of being a physician are enormous, and financial changes, including the influence of managed care, have altered the professional environment. Technology has made practicing medicine more intriguing but also more complicated than ever. Since medical technology has made great advances in medicine possible, our use of it is only likely to expand and develop. Americans value youth, and most of us deny the inevitability of death, thus fostering unrealistic expectations of living forever with the help of technology. With all of these complicated aspects of practicing medicine, addressing emotions is likely not the first thing a physician thinks of when he or she is with patients, nor should it be. There is value to isolating what is physical or biological and having an understanding of the body as separate from the mind. For some aspects of medical practice, emotional detachment is useful and necessary. It could be argued, therefore, that one image of idealized medicine is one in which emotions generally don't get expressed. Although there is a movement in some medical schools across the country to provide more space for students to express their emotions, most doctors probably do not feel that they can talk at length with their colleagues about the emotional challenges of being a doctor or the general emotional difficulties of life.

Given this backdrop, it's also understandable that patients' emotions would not be a primary concern for some physicians. Addressing emotions in patients is discouraged by time constraints, by the scientific principles of medicine, and by the challenges associated with practicing modern medicine. Further, addressing emotions adds another layer to the already difficult job physicians do, and it is sometimes not realistic when there are more acute concerns, as we saw with Susan. It is difficult to say how much Susan can change. We have all seen patients like her go on to develop heart disease. This knowledge can make intervening emotionally feel like an exercise in futility. However, relationships can be very powerful, and possibly ongoing attempts by her physician to understand the emotional components of her illness will assist her in making needed behavioral changes.

Addressing emotions not only benefits patients, it may make the work of doctoring more rewarding. Emotional connections with people are at the heart of what makes most of us happy. Feeling more connected to patients may help buffer against the stresses of practicing medicine and may be equally beneficial for both doctor and patient.

REFERENCES

1. Porter R. *Blood and Guts: A Short History of Medicine.* New York: W.W. Norton and Company; 2002.
2. Singer CJ, Underwood EA. *A Short History of Medicine.* New York: Oxford; 1962.
3. Moulyn A. *Mind-Body: A Pluralistic Interpretation of Mind-Body Interaction Under the Guidelines of Time, Space, and Movement.* New York: Greenwood Press; 1991.
4. Watkins A. Mind-body pathways. In: Watkins A, ed. *Mind-Body Medicine: A Clinicians Guide to Psychoneuroimmunology.* New York: Churchill Livingstone; 2007.
5. Zuger A. Dissatisfaction with medical practice. *N Engl J Med.* 2004;350:69–75.
6. Feldman DS, Novack DH, Gracely E. Effects of managed care on physician–patients relationships, quality of care, and the ethical practice of medicine. *Arch Intern Med.* 1998;158:1626–1632.
7. Donelan K, Blendon RJ, Lundberg GD, et al. The new medical marketplace: physicians' views. *Health Aff (Millwood).* 1997;16:139–148.
8. Heuston WJ. Family physicians satisfaction with practice. *Arch Fam Med.* 1998;7:242–247.
9. Linsk JA. American medical culture and the health care crisis. *Am J Med Qual.* 1993;8:174–180.

10. Bhargava R. *What happened.* London: BMJ Publishing Group. http://bmj.bmjjournals.com/cgi/eletters/322/7294/DC2; 2001 Accessed 15.06.05

11. Eisenberg DM, Davis RB, Ettner SL, et al. Trends in alternative medicine use in the United States, 1990–1997. *JAMA.* 1998;280:1569–1575.

15. Astin JA. Why patients use alternative medicine. *JAMA.* 1998;279:1548–1553.

16. Ogden J, Bavalia K, Bull M. "I want more time with my doctor": a quantitative study of time and the consultation. *Fam Pract.* 2004;21:479–483.

17. Mechanic D, McAlpine DD, Rosenthal M. Are patients office visits with physicians getting shorter? N Engl J Med. 2001;344:198–204.

18. Gabbard GO, Menninger RW. *Medical Marriages.* Washington, DC: American Psychiatric Association; 1988.

3

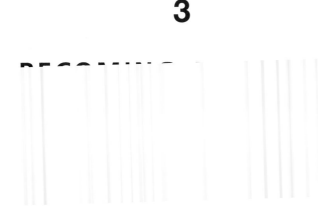

"Health is not valued till Sickness comes."

—Thomas Fuller

Although inevitable, sickness is an unwelcome surprise. There are wide variations in how we cope with illness. This chapter will consider the range of responses to becoming ill. How patients experience illness depends on a variety of disease-specific factors as well as individual patient variables. These individual patient variables involve a number of psychosocial factors including premorbid psychological symptoms; personality factors; and the quality of interpersonal relationships, social support, and financial resources.

Consider the following case examples:

> Steve is a 54-year-old single male who woke up one morning unable to move. He was unable to use the phone to call for help. After yelling for about 3 hours he successfully got the attention of a neighbor to help him. I met him in the hospital a few days later as he was beginning acute rehabilitation for his cerebrovascular accident (CVA). He was extremely anxious and, although eager to talk, reminded me repeatedly that he really didn't need my help; he was just trying to please the staff by talking with me. Rehabilitation staff were unsure whether Steve would regain his ability to walk. However, he left the hospital in a walker, with severe left-sided weakness and mild left neglect.

Jan is a 58-year-old married female who also suffered a CVA. A few days preceding her stroke, she had a myocardial infarction; she had a short hospital stay and was discharged. A few days later she was walking with her husband and collapsed while smoking a cigarette. I met her in the hospital a few days later. She was bright-eyed, pleasant to talk to, and frequently made jokes, which was surprising given that she couldn't walk. She completed acute rehabilitation over the next several weeks and left the hospital in a wheelchair still unable to walk, due to severe left-sided weakness in her lower extremity.

I followed both Steve and Jan while they were inpatients and then as outpatients over the next few years. Although they had similar physical presentations and some very similar aspects in their psychosocial history, the way they coped with their illness and disability was remarkably different. As a result, they had very different outcomes. We will return to Steve and Jan throughout the chapter to illustrate examples of adaptive and nonadaptive coping.

FROM PERSON TO PATIENT: BECOMING ILL

The diagnosis of a serious illness changes lives. Those of us who are healthy take our health for granted. A brief personal example will illustrate this point. A few years ago I was running with my dog on a poorly maintained trail in a park. My dog, quite eager to run that day, saw something of interest and ran faster. As he pulled on the leash, I lost my footing and tripped on a tree root. I fell and, in addition to being scraped on both of my legs, had a severe right ankle injury. It was never clear whether I sustained an avulsion fracture or a grade three sprain. X-rays and a CT scan were inconclusive. Once I wasn't a surgical candidate, the orthopedic specialist became less involved in my care. I was left uncertain of my diagnosis to wait for my ankle to heal. I spent just over 3 months in a cast and spent months after that in physical therapy regaining my previous function. In the spectrum of illnesses that I see patients deal with on a day-to-day basis, this was not a serious injury, but the disruption in my life was enormous. I couldn't drive; I walked with crutches, and, at first, when I was not managing my crutches well, used a wheelchair to see patients in the hospital. Although a relatively benign injury in many ways, I was surprised at the range of feelings I had. I was struck by how I missed things that I had taken for granted such as driving, exercising, and wearing high heels. Though I rarely wear high heels, knowing that I couldn't wear them bothered me. As I recall the injury, I almost never think about the pain I was in; what I remember is the inconvenience, the reaction ...

...ing emotional implications as well.

There is an old saying among physicians and staff who work with brain-injured patients: In terms of personality functioning, a brain injury exacerbates what was there before. For example, if a woman was mean and irritable premorbidly, then she is likely to be more mean and irritable after a brain injury. If she was kind and compliant, she is likely to be more so. This is also somewhat true for persons diagnosed with a serious illness: existing coping patterns and personality factors, whether adaptive or maladaptive, are used during the stress of illness. Though there is tremendous variation among individual coping styles and personalities, there are also common themes that most everyone diagnosed with illness experiences. I will address some the major issues that arise in the context of getting diagnosed with a serious illness and will address variations in coping strategies as well as illustrate coping patterns that are problematic for patients.

THE DIAGNOSTIC PROCESS

For persons who work in medicine, the routine processes of history taking and examination often go unremarked. For the person who is becoming a patient, these processes are anything but routine. Patients are subject to an inherent loss of privacy. Suddenly they are being physically examined by one or more persons who are often not well known to them. In academic institutions, patients are seen by an array of attending physicians, as well as physicians in training. They are required to answer questions about their health and health behaviors. Answering these latter questions can cause patients to feel ashamed. Patients who smoke, who have drug histories, or who have ignored health problems often are embarrassed to tell their doctors about the ways they have not taken care of their bodies. Steve and Jan illustrate these points:

Steve hadn't been to a physician in over 30 years. In my initial contact with him, he often brought this up with everyone he met. He would say, "I knew I had this coming. I should have gone to the doctor." He later told me that he was actually quite aware of his untreated hypertension as he had frequent "high blood pressure headaches." He felt guilty and ashamed about this, and his telling his doctors and staff about this in rehabilitation seemed to be a way of addressing his guilt as well as avoiding feeling uncomfortable with staff, as he imagined they were thinking about his neglect of his body. In the months and years following his hospitalization, Steve never missed a doctor appointment. In fact, he became quite compulsive about his medical appointments and followed up with his outpatient physicians in a very proactive way.

Jan had also not taken care of her body. She was a heavy smoker, was overweight, was a heavy drinker, and she used illegal drugs occasionally. Though she knew she had cardiovascular disease prior to her CVA, she continued smoking. When doctors asked her while in acute rehabilitation about her health behaviors, she looked down and spoke in a barely audible voice. She looked ashamed. She appeared to feel guilty, but in contrast to Steve, was overwhelmed by her guilt. She never talked with anyone about her difficulty taking care of her body and appeared to feel "caught" and exposed by her stroke. In the months and years following rehabilitation, she was sporadic about attending doctor appointments, frequently allowing her husband and family to be in charge of appointment scheduling and outpatient follow-up.

Steve and Jan illustrate the vastly different responses to shame and guilt about not taking care of their bodies. Steve managed his guilt by becoming compulsive about his future medical care, a strategy that worked well for him. It seemed that he was able to allow his doctors to become a part of him in a way that helped him to take better care of himself. This was illustrated by his mentioning his doctors often when speaking with me. When he made decisions about different activities, he often thought about how his doctors would feel about it. Jan, in contrast, never talked about her doctors. She didn't like going to doctor appointments and often "forgot" about her appointments. This forgetting didn't appear to be neurological; she remembered other appointments she had with friends and family. She did not want her physicians to be a part of her life. In fact, she often stated that she wanted to be "left alone."

Another aspect of the diagnostic process involves the use of diagnostic tests. Most people get diagnosed with a serious illness as outpatients. Unlike Steve and Jan, they are fortunate enough not to have a dramatic

They are necessary to work up a patient and provide answers to diagnostic questions; they can dictate the treatment. Many of these tests are physically intrusive and uncomfortable. Patients often forget about the physical discomfort associated with tests, but they remember the physical and psychological intrusion. Although we often do not stop to think about it, it is not normal for us to have scopes and needles placed in our body. One patients expressed his thoughts as follows about a bronchoscopy:

> "It was horrible. They stuck this probe down my throat and I felt like I couldn't breathe. I kept coughing. I think I made the doctor mad. I don't want one of those again."

Notice that this patient didn't even mention the potential diagnostic benefit of the procedure. He was more focused on the physical intrusion associated with the procedure, as well as the worry that he made his doctor angry. This illustrates another point that is especially important during the diagnostic phase of illness: patients worry a lot about making their physician angry. Patients worry that an angry physician won't take care of them. Although I don't think I have ever heard a physician articulate being angry with a patient, especially for something such as not tolerating a procedure, patients think a lot about pleasing their doctors. This is in part related to the nature of being ill. Being sick makes people vulnerable. Some people become very angry about this vulnerability (This will be addressed in Chap. 4); most patients experience anxiety about illness and often react to this anxiety by trying to be good patients. Additionally, vulnerability makes patients realize that they need the doctor. Most people realize that alienating a doctor through anger is not a good way to get help.

Becoming ill changes the routines of daily life. The rote activity of going to work, for example, changes because work is interrupted by a new regimen of doctor appointments, diagnostic tests, and treatment regimens. Almost every patient I see who is recently diagnosed with an illness comments on how much time they spend "at the doctor." This sudden immersion into the medical world is not something most people are prepared for. While many patients can take this on and manage their feelings about being ill and needing the help of physicians, others get overwhelmed.

NORMATIVE AND MALADAPTIVE ANXIETY IN THE FACE OF ILLNESS

Although many people assume that anxiety is negative, anxiety is a normal part of the human experience. Our bodies are equipped with the sympathetic nervous system, in which physiological arousal lets us know when we are upset or that we may be in danger. This is an integral part of the fight/flight response, which we need in order to survive. Anxiety as a response to illness, especially a serious illness, is normal. Furthermore, since anxiety is a normal part of life, most people have developed coping strategies to deal with it. These coping strategies can be adaptive or maladaptive. Maladaptive coping strategies usually intensify in response to the stress of illness. Managing anxiety in an adaptive way often manifests as writing questions down before doctor appointments or bringing supportive friends and family to appointments so they can have help remembering what is being said. Healthy responses to anxiety in response to illness often involve seeking out social support, trying to develop a friendly relationship with the doctor, and following treatment recommendations. Steve's reactions illustrate these points:

Steve managed his anxiety while in the hospital by being friendly with staff. The rehabilitation staff enjoyed working with him and appreciated his sense of humor. While Steve later acknowledged to me that he became friendly with the staff to avoid thinking about how devastated he was, this approach was successful as the relationships he developed maximized his performance in rehabilitation, increased his social support, and kept him from getting too depressed.

While many patients are able to respond to their anxiety productively, anxiety is overwhelming for some patients. Some people who are overwhelmed by anxiety have trouble developing good relationships with their doctors. When anxiety is overwhelming, people have trouble soothing themselves; this makes it difficult to connect with others. Sometimes this can result in alienating those th

Patients who are overwhelmed by anxiety are unsure of whom to trust. Although intense anxiety can result in suspiciousness and paranoia, what I am describing is not paranoia per se, but rather a sense of wanting to be alone to better manage the anxiety. Intense anxiety can cause a sense of hypervigilance, which is the sense that one must keep an eye on everything to prevent something bad from happening. Patients often become hypervigilant following an ICU stay. One man, who had recently been transferred to the floor after a lengthy ICU stay, articulated this by saying, "Every time someone comes near me I think they are going to cause me pain. I feel like I have to watch what is going on all of the time." When patients are hypervigilant, having a lot of contact with medical providers is excruciating because there is a lot of external stimuli to keep track of. Hypervigilant patients often try to figure out what others are thinking. Obviously, it is impossible to know what others are thinking, which leaves hypervigilant patients constantly trying to figure things out, as well as on their guard as they monitors external events. When they are alone, they do not have to do this. This may explain Jan's withdrawal from the rehabilitation staff and her subsequent avoidance of her doctors.

THE NARCISSISTIC INJURY OF ILLNESS

Those of us who are born healthy expect our bodies to work properly. Although this is often overlooked, we all have important relationships with our bodies. Whether we think of ourselves as too fat or thin, too tall or short, having a big nose, or having hair that is too curly, all express an emotional relationship with the bodies that we possess. Some people spend a lot more time thinking about their bodies than others. We all know people who spend a great deal of time thinking about how they can improve their bodies, even though we may think they look fine. The popularity of cosmetic surgery is an example of how seriously many people take their looks. Another aspect of our relationship to our body is how we use it. We expect our bodies to allow us to move around, perform athletically, do our jobs, provide us with sexual pleasure, and allow us to get out of bed effortlessly every morning. Normal aging as well as illness can cause us to loose the ability to function in the way we are used to. For example, people who have spent much of their lives as athletes describe frustration and disappointment at not being able to perform as they are accustomed to as they age. Injury or illness makes this even more difficult. For example, a colleague who has been athletic most of his life and who has been struggling with a chronic shoulder injury talked about not being able to use his body to feel a "rush" after a strenuous workout. For most people, the losses associated with decreased functioning are difficult, but being able to acknowledge those losses helps to ease the blow. We often think of narcissism in pathological terms. A narcissist is someone who is self-centered, grandiose, lacks empathy, and who views relationships in terms of how the relationship is beneficial to him or her. What I am describing is not narcissism in pathological terms, but rather a normal form of narcissism. Not only do we all need some narcissistic qualities to function in the world, our relationship with our body is inherently narcissistic. We learn from a young age that our bodies are capable of great things and our relationship to our body is obviously self-centered. Thinking about our body often doesn't involve another person (although we can bring people into this dialogue such as when we need people to tell us our looks are okay), and we expect that our body is there to serve us. Although it is normal and inevitable that our body will break down and reduce its functional capabilities, we are often surprised when this happens, even if we know intellectually that this is normal. When the body breaks down it is a loss, and for many it is a blow to the ego. We become so accustomed to a working body that adjusting to a body that has reduced capacity is difficult. For some people, this disappointment can lead to profound feelings of devastation. Steve and Jan illustrate the impact of bodily loss.

Steve worked in as a manager of a department store before his stroke. He was on his feet much of the day, and he often helped employees with stocking and shelving. His use of his body was most pronounced in his sexuality, however. Steve did not have a regular romantic relationship, but enjoyed having sex with different

low-level depression that manifested as apathy, boredom, and sleepiness. He was eager to use therapy to help him cope.

Before her stroke, Jan worked as an interior designer, a job that was very demanding on her body. She took a tremendous amount of pride in her ability to make things beautiful and loved being involved in the details of moving furniture, painting, etc. Like Steve, this loss resulted in a chronic depression. Although this depression probably had an organic component, she felt "lost" without her work. This was especially pronounced because although she was married, her marriage was reportedly unfulfilling. She also participated in outpatient therapy to get help with her depression, but she found it difficult to talk with me, stating that she imagined that I wanted "something she was unable to give." She felt empty inside and had no idea how to even begin a discussion about her life or her illness.

Feeling empty is sometimes a response to the narcissistic injury of illness. Patients who excessively fill their lives with work, sex, or even athleticism, can feel empty in response to illness. When they are forced to stop using their bodies, they must rely on their minds for stimulation and comfort. Some people are not accustomed to this and need help relying on their minds in addition to their bodies. This emptiness can lead to chronic depression, as well as anxiety, as some patients become panicked and scared in response to suddenly having time available to be aware of what they are thinking. An important distinction between Steve and Jan was that although Steve felt empty, he was able to use therapy and his other relationships to create a sense of self as well as a sense of meaning about what happened to him. In contrast, Jan's sense of emptiness was related to her increasing isolation. She also became quite resentful of anyone who was physically well and resented her need for therapy to help her cope. In other words, while Steve was able to use therapy to temporarily replace his emptiness, Jan's emptiness was filled up by anxiety and envy, which made benefiting from therapy difficult.

Another aspect of normal narcissism as it relates to our bodies is the extent to which we expect to control what goes on inside of us. Illness reflects a loss of control. When people get sick, they not only have to realize that they must relinquish control to others in order to receive care but they also need to come to terms with the fact that they cannot control what is happening inside of them. One way that many people (both healthy and ill) manage anxiety as it relates to a loss of control is through worrying about getting certain diseases. The most powerful example of this is cancer. Cancer seems to be the illness that most people fear. In popular culture there are all kinds of news stories about which new carcinogen to fear. Especially in the middle and upper-middle classes, people spend a great deal of time consuming organic food or not allowing their children to eat food with artificial colors and preservatives. There is nothing wrong with being mindful of the health risks associated with carcinogens, but the intense fear of cancer has always struck me as a bit odd because more people die of heart disease every year than they do of cancer. I think one reason for the fear of cancer is that the imagery of cancer creates a powerful anxiety that on some level we can all relate to. Simply put, cancer is the body turning on itself. Bad cells emerge, seemingly out of nowhere, and begin to relentlessly attack the good cells. Cancer evokes imagery of good versus evil that takes place beyond our control. Heart disease does not strike up this imagery. People rarely talk about being worried that their heart will stop or that an artery will become blocked. This is in sharp contrast to worries about cancer, in which people can more easily imagine their bodies developing bad cells that will attack what is good inside of them. Fears of cancer reflect a kind of ultimate loss of control, but in any illness loss of control is an important dynamic.

Of course, in reality, our control of our bodies is often illusory. For example, although we do have some control over heart rate and respiration (through relaxation, meditation, or exercise), we can't control the fact that our heart beats and we continue to breathe. These things happen automatically. Illness reminds us of how little control we do have. Some patient's respond to this is by attempting to control what is happening outside of them. This can manifest itself in a number of ways. In the hospital, nurses sometimes complain that certain patients try to "micromanage" their care. Patients may ask several times which medications they are taking or watch nurses or house staff with close scrutiny when they are doing a procedure to make sure they are "doing it right." D

DENIAL OF ILLNESS

Illness can get discovered in one of two ways. For patients like Steve and Jan, acute events occur and are followed by an immediate trip to the hospital. Although the event is acute and the discovery of the illness is dramatic and sudden, it is usually indicative of an underlying chronic disease. The second and more common way illness is diagnosed is through outpatient visits to the doctor and through the insidious onset of physical problems. A patient has symptoms that motivate a visit to the doctor, or abnormal findings on routine exams alert the physician to a problem. Although there are important differences between the two ways illness gets diagnosed, there are a number of similarities regarding the emotional issues that need to be mastered. One of these issues is the extent to which a patient accepts the illness. Upon learning of an illness, shock and disbelief are normal responses. Patients describe this in a variety of ways:

> "I felt like I was in a dream. I saw his mouth moving [the physician's] but I couldn't understand the words. I heard nothing he said about what treatment I should have. I had to call the office a few days later and see if he would tell me again." [A 45-year-old woman diagnosed with breast cancer.]
> "I thought it was a joke at first. He told me I'd have to stick myself with a needle all the time to check my blood sugar. I thought, there is no way in hell I'm going to do that." [A 51-year-old man diagnosed with diabetes.]

Despite the initial normative reactions of shock and disbelief, patients are expected to take their medication and adhere to treatment recommendations. Many people do follow through with treatment recommendations. The man quoted above with Type II diabetes radically overhauled his diet, was medication compliant, and achieved stable control of his glucose levels. However, not all patients follow recommendations provided by their doctors. Even more curious are patients who have signs of serious disease but do not seek medical attention. A patient once described how she had a malignant head and neck growth for over two years before she went to the doctor:

> "It started out as a little bump behind my ear, just the tiniest bump. I felt it in the shower. I tried to forget about it. It got bigger and sometimes I felt it, but I just said to myself, 'This is nothing.' When it got so big that other people could see it, I couldn't hide it anymore. I went to the doctor and he told me I had cancer."

I asked this woman if she was surprised when her doctor told her she had cancer. She smiled wryly and said, "No." This particular patient was quite attractive and a major part of her identity was associated with her looks. I later found out that part of her fear in getting medical attention was that she would have surgery to her head and this would affect her looks. Ironically, it turned out that because she had waited so long to consult her physician about her tumor, the surgery required to resect the tumor left her with disfiguring scars.

It is a curious fact of human nature that we often act in ways that we know intellectually are irrational. Denial is such a process. Patients who are in denial are aware on some level of the fact that they are ill, yet they behave as if they are not. These patients are often successful at convincing themselves that they are well, even when overwhelming evidence would suggest otherwise. Since people have very unique responses to illness, it is difficult to generalize regarding the reasons patients use denial. One common feeling, however, in those who use denial, is paralyzing fear. Illness makes people scared, although there is a lot of variation in the kind of fears people have. Some people are afraid of death; others are afraid of being vulnerable, or being dependent, and so on. One common theme of pathological denial is that the denial is detrimental physically and psychologically to the patient. For both Steve and Jan, denial was an important aspect of their illness.

Before his stroke, Steve consistently ate a poor diet and knew that the food he was eating was not good for him, although he was only minimally overweight. He knew he had high blood pressure because of frequent "high blood pressure headaches." He said that he was able to "put away" his thoughts about having high blood pressure through distracting himself at work or keeping himself busy at home.

further health problems.

Although I have been painting a negative picture of denial, denial is not always bad, particularly if it is brief and prevents being emotionally overwhelmed.[1,2] Studies of persons with cancer, for example, suggest that short-term denial is adaptive and allows people gradually to adjust to the reality of their illness. Steve illustrates the adaptive aspects of denial:

Although Steve was dramatically pushed out of denial following his stroke, he continued to have some denial that served to be adaptive to him. When his neurologist told him that he would be disabled following his stroke, he said to himself, "That's not true, I'll show you." He did exceptionally well in all of his rehabilitation therapies, and in rounds the staff commented on how hard Steve worked and followed suggestions provided by staff. The staff teased him by saying that it was because he was so "stubborn" he was determined to prove them wrong about being disabled, by becoming as functional as possible.

Steve's stubbornness was an important part of his personality. Though it kept him from seeing a doctor in time to prevent his cardiovascular disease, it also helped him to maximize his physical rehabilitation. In the early years of Steve's psychotherapy with me, he often told me that he thought he was in denial. Ironically, the fact that he was so worried about this provided evidence that he was not in as much denial as he thought. Steve was not pathologically denying his illness, but the denial he did have allowed him to get around as he did before his CVA. For example, he laboriously walked up three flights of stairs to my office, which at the time was in an old Victorian building. This not only reflected his desire to get help through psychotherapy but also was related to his desire to prove to himself that he wasn't disabled. He also continued to cook, which was something he loved, despite having only minimal use of his left hand. Although he qualified to have in-home help to prepare his meals, he refused this, stating that he could manage on his own. In fact, as he became less depressed, he threw dinner parties for friends, which gave him a tremendous amount of satisfaction. After many years of therapy, Steve did come to terms with the loss of his functioning and was able to admit that he was disabled. The denial that he had in the first couple of years following his stroke, however, allowed him to avoid a disabling depression and helped him maintain important social contacts.

DEPENDENCY AND ILLNESS

We have seen that denial can be adaptive or pathological; this is also true of dependency. Being ill requires patients to navigate changes in how much they need others to help them. Obviously, this largely depends on the type of illness one has. For example, a patient with fibromyalgia may need to learn to tell her friends when she can't keep up as she used to due to fatigue, while a patient who has a neurological disease may need to learn to tolerate having someone help him bathe. Although there are wide ranges of adjustments required depending on the type of illness, there are common themes of dependency in illness. The first obvious issue relates to patient's need to depend on their doctors. For previously healthy people, illness requires an immersion into a new world in which doctors and ancillary staff are central. Patients have very little choice in this. Although it is true that some patients do strike out on their own and abandon Western medicine altogether in favor of alternative therapies, most patients rely on Western medicine for treatment. The implications of this are both obvious and subtle. A patient who has a job in which other people come for appointments or who has a powerful position suddenly finds himself or herself waiting in physician waiting rooms to be seen at someone else's convenience. Since physicians have the expertise to determine treatment plans, patients cannot determine their own treatment. While this is obvious, this fact is difficult for some patients. For example, occasionally I do presurgical evaluations for situations in which the surgeon has concerns about operating on a particular patient. One woman I saw needed surgery to repair degenerative discs. She was highly ambivalent and continually pressed the surgeon for explanations regarding why the surgery was needed. The surgeon had had several consultation appointments with the patient, yet the patient continued to question the need for surgery. Although it is normal to have a fair amount of anxiety

could just perform the surgery herself. She emphatically agreed and said that performing her own surgery would be easier because she could make sure it "got done right." In some ways this is a variation of a narcissistic injury as the patient was disappointed that she couldn't control all aspects of her surgery. But it also illustrates the difficulties some patients have with relying on others. Especially for people who grew up in homes where they needed to be extremely self-reliant, needing people to help them can cause them to feel terrified because they can't guarantee that something won't go wrong or that the physician will constantly be looking out for them.

Becoming ill or disabled creates a dependence on help from physicians but also from others. Being in a position of suddenly needing others requires a major adjustment for some people. Steve and Jan illustrate important variations in adapting to being more dependent:

Steve was the kind of person who relied on no one else but himself to get through life. He always attempted to appear happy when around other people. As a result of his seemingly persistent good mood he was well liked. He had many acquaintances and a few close friends, although no one close to him ever knew when he was having a difficult time. In his life he had had very few long-term romantic relationships as he always found flaws in persons he dated. His difficulty in relying on others was likely connected to his inability to seek medical attention when it was clear to him that his blood pressure was elevated. While it could be argued that his problems with dependency kept him from having a satisfying emotional life prior to his stroke, it was after his stroke that his difficulty depending on people became something he noticed and considered a problem. For example, Steve had progressed to the point of using a four-point cane to move around. Despite this, he moved slowly, and when he was out it took considerable navigation to cross the street. It was especially difficult for him to get up and down curbs. When he was with friends, and appeared to have difficulty they would offer to help him. This made him extremely angry. He told me that although he realized the good intentions on the part of his friends, he would harshly say, "I can do it myself." He realized that his response was inappropriate and felt guilty for his reactions. Further discussion of these incidents illuminated the fact that although he felt resentful that he needed help, he also had no previous context for getting help. Not only was he self-sufficient as an adult, he grew up in a large family with over-worked and exhausted parents, in which he was largely left to his own devices to care for himself. He began working at the age of 12 and had provided for himself most of his life. It took him a long time to get used to the idea that he didn't have to do everything alone.

Before her stroke, Jan was a very social person. She had many friends and was always busy. Although the rehabilitation staff initially liked Jan, they noticed that at times she behaved quite helplessly. In fact, it seemed to the staff that Jan thought she couldn't do anything for herself. She had good use of her arms and her executive functioning was neurologically unaffected. Yet, her physical and occupational therapists commented that working with Jan was difficult because she seemed to be waiting for them to do the tasks that Jan herself was expected to do. Her progress was not what staff had hoped for. While working with Jan as an outpatient, I found out that her mother had been quite physically ill during most of Jan's childhood. Jan spent a lot of time caring for her mother and it was unclear if there was an adult around who saw to Jan's needs. Jan eventually articulated that she didn't mind being taken care of. In fact, it seemed at times that despite her highly independent background, she felt relieved on some level about finally being cared for. Although this feeling was understandable, her comfort with being cared for likely prevented her from achieving a maximum level of independence in terms of her activities of daily living.

These two dramatically different stories illustrate the impact of not being accustomed to depending on others. Steve's refusal to depend on others ultimately led to his stroke. Despite this, Steve was able to recognize that this was a problem and it was something he actively addressed in psychotherapy. While in the hospital he acknowledged that he "hated" having to receive the help he was receiving. He eventually became more comfortable accepting help from friends, although he negotiated a system with his friends in which they agreed to wait for him to ask for help so that he could ask for assistance on his own when he felt he needed it. Steve also grew used to having his friends pick up items for him at the grocery store and to getting help with household tasks. In contrast, Jan did not feel that the way she was coping was a problem. Her helplessness took over, and she became increasingly dependent on others. Her friends and husband became

also involves accepting emotional loss. No matter what age people are, illness is often experienced as an unfair and unwelcome intrusion. There are certain aspects of illness that need to be mastered and controlled. These aspects of mastery can be likened to developmental phases, and it is important that patients master anxiety and the normative narcissistic injury of illness. They need to avoid pathological denial; yet utilizing some denial can be helpful, especially in the initial phases of illness. Finally, they need to come to terms with the fact that illness causes dependency (although the amount of dependency varies based on the type of illness) and need to become accustomed to accepting help and trusting the doctors they have chosen to provide their care. The different outcomes for Steve and Jan illustrate the importance of mastering these issues:

Steve remained in therapy for several years. He never improved physically despite many subsequent attempts in physical therapy. He continued to have a good relationship with his primary physician and he was compliant with all aspects of his care. He finally came to terms with the idea of himself as disabled. Once he accepted this he became more active. He became involved in a volunteer program in which he worked with hospital patients. He was an admired part of the volunteer staff and became known for his ability in working with "difficult patients." He never became romantically involved although he developed other close friendships that were gratifying. He understood his stroke as an unfortunate event that he could have prevented but appreciated his illness because it helped him to appreciate "what's really important in life."

Jan remained in therapy for a couple of years but never was able to begin a genuine dialogue about her illness and how it affected her. Her helplessness, sadness, and resentment were overwhelming, and she decided that she would be fine "on her own." She went on to develop several other medical problems and became increasingly disabled.

Although there are initial emotional obstacles to be overcome when illness arises, the outcomes of Steve and Jan illustrate the importance of developing a sense of meaning in response to illness. Although we can predict risks for illness based on health behaviors, illness still is and often feels to patients to be a random and unfair occurrence. How patients come to terms with this and understand this is a crucial aspect of dealing with the impact of becoming a patient. As we will see in the next chapter, developing a sense of meaning about one's illness is intimately tied to the emotional and psychological well-being of patients who are recovering from and coping with a serious or chronic illness.

REFERENCES

1. Greer S. The management of denial in cancer patients. *Oncology* 1992; 6(12):33–36.
2. Matt DA, Sementilli ME, Burish TG. Denial as a strategy for coping with cancer. *J Mental Health Counsel.* 1988; 10(2):136–144.

4

"We are perhaps, uniquely among the earth's creatures, the worrying animal. We worry away our lives, fearing the future, discontent with the present, unable to take in the idea of dying, unable to sit still."
                                                        —Lewis Thomas

Adjusting to illness requires patients to accept loss, manage the blow to the ego that illness causes, cope with anxiety, and manage feeling more dependent. Although the issues discussed in Chapter 3 may be present when an illness is either acute or chronic, there are unique psychological challenges that arise after active medical treatment, when illness becomes chronic, and also in some cases when patients are physically asymptomatic and recovering from an illness. The challenges that arise after active medical treatment and the psychological consequences of chronic medical problems are the focus of this chapter.

Many patients who are diagnosed with an illness and are involved in active medical treatment have a marked absence of psychiatric symptoms. While there are exceptions to this, for example, if a patient cannot successfully manage the dynamics of acute illness as described in Chapter 3, most patients are not overwhelmed with emotional problems during active treatment. Additionally, even if a patient has not been able to manage the issues caused by acute illness, the physical demands of illness often take precedence over psychological demands during medical treatment. In many cases, patients are simply too ill to be preoccupied with worry or anxiety. There is a saying in hospitals that when patients get irritable it's time for them to be discharged. This makes sense because being in the hospital is for the most part an unpleasant experience. When patients are really ill, they tend not to notice the unpleasant aspects of hospitalization, but when they are better they are likely to get annoyed and want to leave. Being less focused on physical problems allows more psychological energy to focus on emotional problems. Additionally, when patients are acutely ill, health care professionals, as well as family and friends often surround patients in the active phase of medical treatment. The social support of such individuals around the patient can often buffer the patient from depression and anxiety. After active medical treatment however, patients often get less social support, much in the way that persons who experience the death of a loved one report that after the funeral friends and extended family go back to their own lives, while they are left to deal with the intense emotions that arise, usually with less psychosocial support.

As a result of the above factors, it is often after active medical treatment that patients are extremely vulnerable to anxiety, depression, and even psychosomatic experiences. Many patients articulate that they feel more helpless after medical treatment when nothing is being done to them to treat their disease. Further, some patients become quite dependent on contact with their health care professionals. While this contact can have multiple meanings for patients, many patients say that they develop a sense of security when around medical staff. When this contact stops, some patients get scared that they will become sick and that no one will be around to help them. It is during this time that patients often report terrifying worries of being reinjured, of having recurrences of their original disease, or of developing another disease that is completely unrelated to their original illness.

The patients I will be describing fall into one of two categories. The first group consists of patients who receive treatment for a serious illness (often a malignancy) and are in remission. They have no signs of symptoms of disease and often resume some semblance of their normal functioning. The second group consists of those patients who, after treatment, are left with chronic symptoms.

RESUMING LIFE AFTER A SERIOUS ILLNESS

Consider the following case example:

cleared to go back to work part-time. Robin attempted to resume work, but found that when she went to work, she couldn't concentrate. She wasn't excited about work in the way she had been in the past and noted that she felt numb and detached. She said she felt most comfortable when she was at home watching television or reading a book. When I asked Robin how she was sleeping at night, she told me that she got very anxious around bedtime and that when she did sleep she had dreams about "dying animals." These dreams were very disturbing, and she often avoided sleep by watching television or surfing the Internet.

One way to think about a serious illness is that it is a traumatic event. The fourth edition of the *Diagnostic and Statistical Manual of Mental Disorders* for the first time characterized a life-threatening illness as a traumatic event. This has resulted in a number research articles regarding the prevalence of post-traumatic stress disorder (PTSD) in medically ill populations. Much of this research has been conducted with cancer patients, and although the research has yielded inconsistent results, initial data suggests that a significant proportion of cancer patients experience PTSD or PTSD symptoms, although the percentage of patients with PTSD varies based on study methodology. Additionally, there is a fair amount of controversy within the field regarding how to measure PTSD in cancer patients.[1,2] A recent review article found that in 13 studies the incidence of PTSD occurred in 0 percent to 32 percent of patients following cancer diagnosis and treatment.[3] A prospective study, which is often thought to be a better methodology for research, found that in a group of sixty-three head and neck, and lung cancer patients at six-months following treatment, 22 percent of the patients met criteria for PTSD, and 16 percent of patients had multiple PTSD symptoms.[4]

The other group of medical patients that have been studied with regards to PTSD are those with heart disease. Myocardial infarction (MI) and coronary artery bypass surgery are both experiences that cause patients to fear that they may die and thus can be considered traumatic. A recent review article found that although many patients do well following hospitalization for MI or surgeries for heart-related conditions, a significant minority of patients develop PTSD.[5] Studies cited in this review found that approximately 15 percent of patients who undergo bypass grafting or aortic valve replacement develop PTSD and that 8 percent to 25 percent of patients who have an MI develop PTSD.

The definition of a trauma as described by the 4th edition of the *Diagnostic and Statistical Manual of Mental Disorders* (DSM-IV) is that a person "experienced, witnessed, or was confronted with an event that involved actual or threatened death or serious injury, or a threat to the physical integrity of self or others." The threat also imposes "intense fear, helplessness, or horror."[6] Experiencing a trauma is the first criterion for a diagnosis of post-traumatic stress disorder. Other symptoms of PTSD include intrusive memories, nightmares, a sense of reliving the event, or psychological distress when reminded of the event. Another set of symptoms includes avoidance of thoughts or feelings of the event, inability to recall certain aspects of the event, withdrawal from others, a sense of a foreshortened future, or emotional numbing. Finally, the diagnosis of PTSD also involves two of the following: insomnia, irritability, concentration difficulties, hypervigilance, or an exaggerated startle response. It is probably obvious to the reader that some of the symptoms of PTSD are often a part of what happens to most people as a result of being treated for a serious illness. Concentration problems can result from medical treatments (such as chemotherapy) or medications. This can also be the case with insomnia. Additionally, insomnia is present in almost every hospital patient I have seen and therefore cannot be accurately assessed in hospital inpatients. Persons who are diagnosed with serious illness often fear that their future is shortened, but this is an expected consequence of severe, life-threatening illness. Another issue with the diagnosis of PTSD in medically ill populations is that the experience of illness is often not a discrete event as is true for some other kinds of traumatic events. Illness is often chronic, and patients are subject to long periods of difficult treatments and fear about the impact of their illness and their safety.

While these factors might put the validity of a PTSD diagnosis in med-

intrusive procedures as well as to receive more attention from medical professionals. For example, a patient who goes in for heart surgery and develops complications that results in a long ICU stay is someone who is subjected to far more intrusive medical procedures and the experience of being bombarded by stimuli (nurses, doctors, loud noises from machines in the ICU) than someone who has outpatient chemotherapy for a malignancy. The former situation often results in what I think of a normative stress response from being in the hospital. Such patients often present with hypervigilance, a fear of nurses and physicians, severe anxiety, severe insomnia (usually due to a fear of falling asleep and being startled awake), and difficulty talking about their illness. These patients are often uncomfortable and anxious and often request anxiolytics to help manage their anxiety. Although such patients can be a problem to manage for hospital staff, a diagnosis of PTSD is often not warranted because the symptoms often dissipate as the patient needs less acute care and gets out of the hospital.

Other patients however, like Robin, do go on to develop PTSD. In fact, research suggests that some cancer patients develop PTSD well after their treatment.[4] Patients who develop PTSD in response to a serious illness are overwhelmed. They sometimes have difficulty seeking out psychological help for their symptoms because they will have to talk about their illness. In my experience, this is characteristic of an avoidance symptom that is part of a PTSD diagnosis. Often these patients will be referred for mental health treatment but will not follow through with the referral. The patients that do present for psychological treatment are often those that are bombarded by intrusive memories, thoughts, or nightmares and they realize that getting help could reduce their distress. In Robin's case, she sought out treatment at the insistence of her husband, who was increasingly worried about Robin's isolation and withdrawal. Although Robin was bothered by nightmares, she felt numb during the day and therefore was not very distressed most of the time. When I spoke with her for the first time, however, it became clear that when she did think about her illness she felt overwhelmed. She said,

> "I don't think about it most of the time, and so I feel fine. When I do think about it, I feel as if I can't breathe. I get panicked. All I can think about is that I'll be in the 10 percent that doesn't make it. I find myself thinking about whether I should buy clothes for the spring. I can't imagine that I will live out the rest of my lifespan."

Robin had avoided thinking about her illness because when she did the fear was so intense that she actually felt at times that she could die imminently. Although the feature of impending doom or worry of imminent death is often a feature of panic disorder, I find that in such patients the range of somatic symptoms that can accompany panic disorder does often not accompany the anxiety. Rather, this feeling of imminent death is more like a breakthrough of emotions that have been avoided throughout treatment. In some cases this feeling may be a memory related to events in the hospital. Sometimes, patients who experience this level of symptoms have histories of anxiety that have been managed by working in highly demanding careers. For health professionals, people who work in finance or business, or people who work in executive management careers, the demanding nature of their work prevents anxiety from getting overwhelming as they are constantly distracted by external situations. Although this is similar to using work as a way to not think about emotional issues, such patients are usually aware of their anxiety and actively fight to keep it under control. They may have histories of substance abuse, which is a common way to self-medicate anxiety. Robin illustrates these points:

> Before her diagnosis of cancer, Robin was very high functioning at work. She was also happily married and had a nice home in an area that she loved. Yet, she described that even before she was diagnosed with cancer, she felt "unappreciative" of what she had. She felt troubled much of the time about how unhappy she was and especially now feels guilt about the fact that she

couldn't "appreciate every day." She said that she got irritable with her husband for "little things" and noted that she drank alcohol most nights to
"take the edge off" her irritability and anxiety. Because she had trouble
sleeping, she also used alcohol to help treat her insomnia. About her

her life. She described herself as always being "in control" with friends,
family, and in her marriage. It became clear that Robin avoided thinking
about her illness because she was unable to tolerate the idea that such a
serious illness could take her life. This thought was so difficult for her to
accept that she simply put it out of her mind during the diagnostic and
active treatment phase of her illness. Ironically, once she felt better physically, she lived with the constant threat that she would die.

Robin's sense of living a lie is also a common experience for persons with
PTSD symptoms. Moving on after a traumatic illness involves reemerging
into one's life, which often involves going to work, seeing friends, caring for
children, and so on. Persons who are having trouble integrating the trauma
of illness and have PTSD symptoms, feel as if they are fraudulent or lying
when they allow themselves to enjoy or return to their lives. A sense of living a lie is also connected with an idea that things that used to seem important (such as earning enough money or acquiring possessions) are no
longer as important as they used to be. Some people who have this realization can ultimately feel more satisfied with their lives if these feelings result
in a new or renewed sense of meaning or purpose. Others, however, feel isolated because they have no sense of meaning about what happened to them.
Although illness is often random, patients who develop a story regarding
why they were ill tend to cope better. For example, patients often say that
they think getting sick was a message to slow down or to appreciate the
things that they have. Some patients develop a renewed sense of spirituality or religious involvement. People who cannot develop a sense of meaning regarding their illness, often feel at the mercy of illness and worry that
they will get sick again, either with a recurrence of their original disease or
a new disease. Robin's experiences highlight this dynamic:

As Robin became more aware of her anxiety, she began to worry about becoming HIV positive or getting AIDS. She had no risk factors for contracting HIV and had negative test results when she had been tested in the past. She often requested HIV testing from her physician to reassure herself she was not HIV positive.

Robin illustrates the impact of realizing one's vulnerability on a young person who develops a life-threatening illness. Robin's realization of the random nature of illness caused her to feel hopeless and out of control. Worrying about getting another illness was a way to organize this anxiety and a way to try (though unsuccessfully) to prepare herself for another surprise illness. She could not enjoy herself for fear that letting her guard down would invite the illness to return. Worry in this manner is an attempt to be prepared for the worst.

We often expect that young people have trouble accepting their vulnerability, but this is a common issue in older adults as well. Consider the example of John:

John was fifty-seven when he had an arterial graft repair to stop a life-threatening blockage to his small intestine. He came to psychotherapy six-years later because he frequently presented to his primary care doctor with symptoms of chronic pain. He had no signs of disease and had received extensive diagnostic work-ups. He presented initially as very wary of therapy and felt that since his problems were physical in nature, he did not need help from a psychologist. Although his surgery was six-years prior to our initial meeting he spoke of it as if it had just happened. After meeting with him a few times he told me that his small bowel arterial disease was congenital and discovered "almost accidentally" because his only symptom was nausea when he presented to his primary doctor. If he hadn't had this blockage discovered, he could have died. He interpreted this as a "brush with death" and although he felt lucky to be alive, he constantly worried that something unpredictable could happen again. As he began to understand these worries his psychosomatic symptoms disappeared.

Although ironic, people who manage to get better from a serious illness sometimes develop psychosomatic symptoms. As we saw with Robin, these symptoms are often a reflection of overwhelming fear and difficulty managing thoughts about their illness. In such circumstances, psychosomatic symptoms are also usually intricately tied in with an intense fear of death and vulnerability. In my work with John, it was clear that not only

indicate that they never thought that aging would happen to them! In talking with such patients it seems to be the case that for some, aging is tied in with regrets about what hasn't been accomplished in life, missed opportunities, and a wish to have done things differently. Bring able to think about these things requires a history of being able to cope well with emotions as well as disappointment. Some patients are unable to think about painful and disappointing emotional issues without help.

Patients who have a serious illness need to come to terms with their vulnerability. This involves realizing that their body has failed them, but illness also brings into focus the inevitability of aging and death. How patients have dealt with feeling vulnerability in the past, especially emotionally vulnerable, is usually an indicator of how they will tolerate the vulnerability associated with serious disease.

Some patients who are overwhelmed by vulnerability can develop PTSD symptoms, but all patients are faced with the task of how to resume a normal life after recovering from an illness. Many people do this quite well; they are able to integrate the illness experience into their identity, manage the feelings of fear and vulnerability associated with being ill, and usually come to terms with the limitations of their bodies and the inevitability of mortality. Others have different problems as the nature of illness forces people to confront a variety of issues.

ANGER IN RESPONSE TO ILLNESS

The end of active treatment often creates room for people to worry about illness recurrence or their future. Some people develop anxiety in response to worry and fear; others get angry. They may feel resentful that they became ill, and though an underlying emotion might be paralyzing fear of the illness returning, they present as angry and often complain of feeling misunderstood by those around them. Consider the following case example:

> Susan is a 23-year-old woman who developed a rare cancer during college. She went through treatment, did well, and had a good prognosis. Although she had gone back to school, she was having difficulty adjusting. Susan found herself plagued with fears that her cancer would return and felt alienated by family and friends because they didn't understand her worry about her cancer returning. She felt very angry that they didn't feel more sympathetic to her anxiety and also resentful that others didn't have to worry about developing a life-threatening illness. She said, "I went through cancer treatment and was fighting for my life, and now I am expected to act normal . . . just to be around everyone who is stressed out about finals? I bet I am the only one worried that the stress I have will make me relapse."

Susan's comments illustrate many important issues in persons who undergo treatment for a serious illness. Susan didn't feel normal, and in some ways, she was right. Developing a serious illness when young isn't normal and an additional challenge for young people who develop serious illnesses is to come to terms with this.

Susan's comments also illustrate the common worry about the impact of stress. Many patients, young and old, believe that the stress in their lives caused their disease. This belief often puts patients in a difficult emotional bind: if they are to accept that stress caused their disease, then they feel the need to believe that they did not control their stress appropriately and thus conclude that they are to blame for their illness. Patients who develop a lot of anger following an illness are usually aware of being in this bind. They articulate feeling resentful of popular books that encourage positive feelings in response to one's illness or that suggest that attitude change will reduce the chances of illness recurrence. Susan's comments illustrate the above:

> "The thing I hate most is being told that I have been given a gift by getting cancer, how lucky I should be to appreciate every day. What a joke! I don't appreciate every day, and now I feel guilty about that on top of everything else I'm feeling. If anything, I realize now how hard life is."

Illness takes away one's ability to take life for granted, which is developmentally normal in young people, and this loss is often perceived as unfair and unjust. People who develop a lot of anger in response to having been ill are in a difficult emotional position. People (both

patient to stop feeling resentful and to feel lucky. While these statements are well-intended, patients at times experience this as a denial of what they have been through. I will talk more about family dynamics in Chapter 6.

Some patients develop a lot of anger following the diagnosis and treatment of a serious illness; some anger about being unlucky in becoming ill is normal. Usually if anger is acknowledged and understood by health care professionals, family, or friends, it dissipates and patients do not feel that they are in the position of having to keep justifying their anger. Paradoxically, the more that the angry patients are told to let go of their anger, the angrier they become.

WHEN SYMPTOMS AND LIMITATIONS ARE CHRONIC

Many patients do not get completely better following treatment for medical problems. These patients undergo unique psychological stress that can include lifestyle and vocational alterations to accommodate ongoing symptoms, financial stress due to lost work income, unpredictability regarding physical symptoms, and chronic pain. Though some patients are aware upon the diagnosis of a serious illness that they will have chronic symptoms, many patients are not aware of this. Consider the example of Joe:

> Joe is a 57-year-old who worked in a middle management position in the technology industry. He was diagnosed with a cervical spine disease and needed surgery to repair and fuse several of his vertebrae. At the time I met Joe, he had just undergone his second surgery, as he continued to have neck pain as well as numbing in his hand. He had sought

> out another surgeon for his second surgery, but the second surgery did not relieve his symptoms. During the second year he was in treatment with me, he had a third surgery by yet a different surgeon. The third surgery did not relieve his pain. He eventually became disabled from work. He spoke frequently of feeling "cheated" by all of his doctors. He said, "I always used to think that doctors are supposed to make you better. I just don't understand how I can feel worse. I thought after all this surgery my pain would be gone."

Most of us are taught that doctors make us better. "Better" is often interpreted as pain-free and symptom-free. When this doesn't happen, it is incredibly disappointing for patients who are then vulnerable to both depression and anxiety. In fact, the rates of anxiety and depression are significant in chronically ill populations. Data from the United States National Comorbidity Survey Part II found that in persons reporting any kind of physical disorder in the past year, 31.8 percent reported an anxiety disorder also occurring in the last year. These findings were adjusted for the impact of major depression, sociodemographic factors, and substance use.[7] Rates of depression are also high in chronically ill populations, with rates ranging from 14 percent to 27 percent of heart disease patients, 4 percent to 42 percent of cancer patients, 7 percent to 27 percent of cerebrovascular accident patients, 22 percent of patients with Parkinson's disease, and 10 percent of a community sample of diabetics.[8]

Although anxiety and depression can and do precede illness, as discussed in Chapter 1, anxiety and mood disorders are a consequence of illness, especially when patients have chronic pain. In recent years, increasing attention has been paid to the high prevalence of chronic pain. Studies in major cities across the world have found rates of chronic pain to range from 5 percent to 33 percent.[9] One study of a community sample in Scotland found the rate of self-reported chronic pain as high as 46 percent.[10]

Chronic pain can impact every aspect of people's lives, and persons with chronic pain often have psychological sequelae. While rates of depression in medically ill patients is high, the rates of depression in persons with chronic pain are strikingly so. An estimated 30 percent to 54 percent of clinic-based chronic pain patients meet criteria for major depression.[8] Although many chronic pain patients have affective disorders before the onset of chronic pain, the presence of anxiety or depression does not appear to predict chronic pain in recovery.[11] In other words, it is not clear that anxiety or depression is causal in pain disorders. In fact, depression often follows chronic pain; since pain and depression have similar neuro-

I got to know him, however, it was clear that his life wasn't always so calm. Joe had been addicted to heroin in his early twenties, a period in which his main activities revolved around procuring heroin. After a few years, though, he grew tired of this lifestyle and successfully used methadone to get off heroin permanently. Around this time, he met his wife who was also supportive of his abstaining from using drugs. After his first surgery, Joe was prescribed narcotics for pain. Although he used these responsibly, he became very worried about his potential to abuse them, although there was no evidence that he would do so, in fact, he often forgot to take his medication and frequently tried to get by with minimal doses. I soon understood that Joe's depression resulted not only from chronic pain but that also his from use of narcotics, which reminded him of his past use of heroin. Before his surgery, he had been successful in not thinking about this part of his life, what might have led him to use drugs, as well as the lost time associated with using drugs during his twenties. Once he was reminded of his past through using narcotics for pain control, he became overwhelmed with grief; this seemed to contribute not only to his depression, but also to his intense focus on his pain. While this eventually decreased and Joe was able to improve functioning, he articulated that he felt that his pain was "payback" for all he had done wrong in the past.

While many patients get depressed as a result of pain, and while there may be similar neurochemical pathways between pain and depression that may partially explain these associations, I have found in some cases that depression is intimately linked with past experiences of loss, as well as feelings of guilt and regret. Joe's feeling of being punished through his pain and illness is common. Many patients wonder what they have done to deserve the illness they are experiencing. Often this is a way to try to make sense of their illness as well as to increase a sense of control. Although thinking about what one has done to cause illness is an attempt to develop a sense of meaning, doing so through blaming oneself is usually not helpful and exacerbates depression.

CONCLUSIONS

The end of active medical treatment involves less contact with medical professionals, and many patients develop new psychological symptoms during this phase of illness. The absence of active treatment allows room for worry about illness recurrence and forces patients to face the painful realities of vulnerability and mortality. This can result in both depression and/or anxiety.

Living with chronic illness requires patients to adapt to chronic pain and reductions in functioning and to manage the disappointment that medical treatment has not been able to make them symptom-free. Anxiety and depression are common results of living with chronic medical symptoms, and patients must learn to integrate their illness into their life.

Patients who are recovering from illness or living with illness benefit from having a sense of meaning about what has happened to them. By a "sense of meaning" I do not mean to imply that patients need to adopt a falsely naive or optimistic attitude about their illness. In fact, illness needs to be accepted as a part of who they are. Emotional recovery from illness involves varying degrees of sadness, loss, anger, helplessness, and vulnerability. Patients who cope well emotionally with illness do not ignore these feelings; rather, they integrate them into their identity through thinking about them and talking about them with supportive friends, family, and medical and mental health professionals.

REFERENCES

1. Cordova MJ, Studts JL, Hann DM, Jacobsen PB, Andrykowski MA. Symptom structure of PTSD following breast cancer. *J Trauma Stress.* 2000;13:301–319.
2. DuHamel KN, Ostroff J, Ashman T, et al. Construct validity of the posttraumatic stress disorder checklist in cancer survivors: analyses based on two samples. *Psychol Assess.* 2004;16:255–266.
3. Kangas M, Henry JL, Bryant RA. Posttraumatic stress disorder following cancer: a conceptual and empirical review. *Clin Psychol Rev.* 2002;22:499–524.

4. Kangas M, Henry JL, Bryant RA. The relationship between acute stress disorder and posttraumatic stress disorder following cancer. *J Consult Clin Psychol.* 2005;73:360–364.

5. Doerfler LA, Paraskos, JA. Posttraumatic stress disorder in patients with coro-

diathesis stress framework. *Psychol Bull.* 1996;119:95–110.

9. Gureje O, Von Korff M, Simon GE, Gater R. Persistent pain and well-being: A world health organization study in primary care. *J Am Med Assoc.* 1998;280: 147–152.

10. Elliott AM, Smith BH, Penny KI, Smith WL, Chambers WA. The epidemiology of chronic pain in the community. *Lancet.* 1999;354:1248–1252.

11. Gureje O, Simon GE, Von Korff M. A cross national study of the course of persistant pain in primary care. *Pain.* 2001;92:195–200.

12. Fishbain D, Cutler R, Rossomoff HL, Rossomoff RS. Chronic pain associated depression: antecedent or consequence of chronic pain? A review. *Clin J Pain.* 1997;13:116–137.

5

"*Formerly, when religion was strong and science weak, men mistook magic for medicine; now, when science is strong and religion weak, men mistake medicine for magic.*"

—Thomas Szasz

Medical patients are vulnerable both to anxiety and depression as well as difficulty coping with the chronic nature of illness. Primary care physicians are in a unique position to help patients who become depressed or anxious, as they are likely to have more contact with patients than specialist physicians. Further, clinicians who follow patients over a long period of time are in the unique and important position to recognize changes in patients' mood and psychological symptoms. In addition to providing social support for patients, primary care physicians can also prescribe medications that potentially can alleviate psychological distress. The focus of this chapter is to discuss pharmacological interventions and is intended to address some of the issues encountered by primary care physicians who prescribe psychotropic medications. The emphasis of this chapter is on antidepressants, as these are often first-line agents for both anxiety and depressive disorders. Anxiolytics, such as benzodiazepines will also be discussed. Since medical patients are often on multiple medications, I will address clinically relevant drug interactions involving antidepressants. The chapter will end with a discussion of special concerns regarding agents affecting serotonin.

Primary care physicians are increasingly providing treatment to patients with mental and emotional disorders. In fact, most estimates suggest that the majority of mental health treatment in the United States is provided by primary care clinicians.[1,2] Although there is evidence that primary care clinicians can provide effective pharmacotherapy for more than 75 percent of patients with depression, there is considerable variability in practice as to whether they do prescribe medications for depression, the most common psychiatric disorder seen in outpatient practices.[3,4] This likely is due to a number of factors. First, different clinicians have different comfort levels with diagnosing mental illness. Second, patients may not be open with physicians about their psychological symptoms and histories. Third, physicians may not have the time needed to provide thorough diagnostic evaluations for certain patients, particularly those that have complex medical problems, extensive psychiatric histories, or personality disturbances.

Research suggests that some patients who are prescribed medication for a psychiatric illness in primary care practice do not receive adequate follow-up. Two studies, one in the United States and one in Australia, found that pharmacological antidepressant treatments in primary care settings were either too brief or that dosages were too low.[5,6] Another study that looked at patient discontinuation of antidepressants found discrepancies between instructions that physicians reported having given to patients and patients' recollections of what they were told about duration of treatment as well as adverse side effects.[7] This same study found that when patients had three or more follow-up visits related to their medication that they were more likely to continue antidepressant treatment, thus reinforcing the need for close follow-up once psychotropic medications are prescribed. Close follow-up after prescribing an antidepressant is important because patients often do have side effects to many psychotropic medications. If they are able to meet with their doctor two to four weeks after starting a new medication, they have a chance to ask questions about side effects and to receive reassurance that certain side effects are normal which may decrease the likelihood of discontinuation. Further, such a meeting allows the physician to monitor the medications' efficacy as well as possible serious adverse effects. This model is similar to that which is practiced by many psychiatrists and psychopharmacologists.

It may be true that patients discontinue medication because they do not know how long to remain on an antidepressant (current guidelines for major depressive disorder suggest that patients should remain on medica-

response to antidepressants and only 25 percent to 35 percent experience a complete remission of their symptoms.[9-11] These findings place another burden on physicians and mental health professionals. Patients often have the idea that an antidepressant will take away all of their symptoms. In my experience, when patients achieve only partial reduction in symptoms, some want to stop taking the medication instead of working with their physician to achieve an appropriate dosage, adding another medication, or adding psychotherapy. The reasons for this are likely complicated. First, there is a very strong idea in American culture that we should get better quickly when we are medically ill or suffering. Pharmaceutical companies seem to be aware of this, and their drugs are marketed accordingly. Second, many patients are unprepared for adverse side effects of medication, even if their physician has talked with them about what to expect. Third, many patients are ambivalent about taking antidepressants. They complain that they do not want to add one more medication to their treatment regimen or be dependent on a pill to help their mood. Additionally, some patients who are in psychotherapy do not feel that they need combined treatment (both psychotherapy and medication). There is some validity to this last point as both pharmacological interventions as well as psychotherapy have equal efficacy in the treatment of depression, although combined treatments are probably more efficacious in cases of more severe, recurrent depression.[12-14] It should be noted that one study found that in patients with recurrent depression and histories of childhood trauma, psychotherapy alone was more beneficial than antidepressant monotherapy.[14] Thus, one way to approach this situation is to talk with patients about the risks and benefits of both kinds of treatments and ask them what they prefer. While many patients are reluctant to take psychiatric medication, many patients are equally reluctant to receive psychotherapy. In cases in which a patient prefers medication, the primary care physician can provide pharmacological treatment successfully in many cases. The remainder of this chapter will address pharmacological treatments for depression and anxiety disorders commonly encountered in medical patients. This discussion will be limited, however, to diagnoses of major depressive disorder (MDD), generalized anxiety disorder (GAD), panic disorder (PD), and post-traumatic stress disorder (PTSD), especially PTSD related to medical treatment. Chapter 9 will address guidelines for referral to mental health providers for psychotherapy, as well as when to consult a medication specialist if a patient doesn't respond to pharmacological treatment in the primary care setting.

ANTIDEPRESSANTS FOR MAJOR DEPRESSION

As the reader likely already knows, treating depression is dependent on accurate diagnosis. Table 1 reviews the criteria for major depressive disorder as defined by the fourth edition, text revision of the *Diagnostic and Statistical Manual of Mental Disorders* (DSM-IV-TR).[15] One diagnostic algorithm, developed as a guide for primary care physicians, suggests asking the following two questions to screen for the presence of depression.[16] This approach is also more efficient for busy primary care clinicians. The questions are (1) During the past month, have you been often bothered by feeling down, depressed, or hopeless? (2) During the past month, have you been bothered by having little interest or pleasure in doing things? If the answers to both questions are "no," the patient is unlikely to have MDD. These authors suggest that if the patient answers "yes" to both questions you should proceed with a depression interview.

DSM-IV-TR also has a subtype referred to as atypical depression. Atypical depression involves mood reactivity and two of the following: interpersonal sensitivity, weight gain, hypersomnia, and leaden paralysis. (Leaden paralysis is a heavy feeling in the extremities.) Note that anxious rumination and irritability, which are also listed in Table 1, are symptoms that are commonly seen in depressed patients, but are not required for the diagnosis. It is important to screen for anxiety when evaluating depression symptoms, as the presence of anxiety worsens the outcome of depression.[17] Regarding irritability, it has been found that up to 40 percent of patients with MDD report being irritable more than half of the time.[18]

Table 1. Diagnostic criteria for major depressive disorder (MDD)

Five or more of the following symptoms during the same two-week period:

Depressed mood

Anhedonia

[...text obscured...]

2. Two or more symptoms:

Significant weight gain

Increase in appetite

Leaden paralysis

Pattern of interpersonal sensitivity

Additional common symptoms not required as part of MDD diagnosis but commonly seen in depressed patients

Anxious rumination

Irritability

Initial screening questions

1. During the past month, have you been often bothered by feeling down, depressed, or hopeless?

2. During the past month, have you been bothered by having little interest or pleasure in doing things?

Reprinted with permission from the Diagnostic and Statistical Manual of Mental Disorders, Fourth Edition, Text Revision, (Copyright 2000). American Psychiatric Association.

All antidepressants tend to be comparably efficacious regardless of class for the treatment of major depression.[10,19] Choosing an antidepressant should be based on past patient experiences of medications and side effect profiles. Since selective serotonin reuptake inhibitors (SSRIs) have a low-side effect profile compared to the tricyclic antidepressants (TCAs), SSRIs are often used in the treatment for depression, as are newer antidepressant agents. Because of recent emphasis on both empirically based medical practice as well as a redefinition of the treatment of depression to strive for remission as opposed to response, a number of algorithms have been developed to guide clinicians in the treatment of depression. Perhaps one of the most noteworthy of these algorithms is the Texas Medication Algorithm Project, which evaluated "treatment as usual" versus an algorithm for patients with major depression who had relatively severe symptoms, poor daily functioning, concurrent medical conditions, and alcohol and other substance abuse.[20] The algorithm suggests that in addition to considering SSRIs as initial treatment for depression, other medications that can be considered initially are bupropionSR, nefazadone, venlafaxineXR, or mirtazapine. (Concerns regarding nefazadone and hepatotoxicity have led to an FDA warning regarding this medication, and therefore it should be prescribed cautiously.) It should also be noted that as of the date of this writing, venlafaxine has been found in three metaanalyses to have higher rates of achieving remission as compared with the SSRIs,[21] although most of the literature continues to report that there is no difference in antidepressant efficacy. If only a partial response is achieved with the initial trial, augmentation can be considered, or the patient could be given a trial of another antidepressant. Stage two of the algorithm allows for the use of a TCA, or any of the other medications recommended in the first stage. Monoamine oxidase inhibitors (MAOIs) are recommended after trials of newer antidepressants and a TCA. (While MAOIs are effective in treating depression, patients need to follow a low tyramine diet, which limits their clinical utility.) The rest of the algorithm provides detailed suggestions regarding how to augment antidepressants as well as helpful decision trees. The reader wanting more information is encouraged to view the entire protocol of the Texas Medication Algorithm Project. Access to this information is located in at the end of the chapter.

Clinicians often wonder if once an initial trial of an SSRI fails if it makes sense to try another SSRI, as all SSRIs have the same mechanism of action and similar side effect profiles. There does appear to be a rationale for trying another SSRI if a clinician wishes to use the same class of medications. A leading expert in the field of psychopharmacology, Stephan Stahl, notes that among the SSRIs, individual patients can have very unique responses, thus trying another SSRI may yield a different response.[22] Further, research suggests that 50 percent to 60 percent of patients will respond to a different SSRI after an initial trial has been unsuccessful.[21] Another common question that clinicians have is regarding SSRI discontinuation syndrome, which is a concern with all SSRIs, except fluoxetine, which has a very long half-life. Because of serotonin discontinuation syndrome, all SSRIs except fluoxetine should be tapered off gradually. This is especially true with paroxetine, which has a strong association with withdrawal symptoms.[23] Discontinuation syndrome will be discussed in more detail at the end of the chapter.

...... suggested that adding a benzodiazepine with an antidepressant should be considered in patients who are not at risk for benzodiazepine-related adverse effects. This recommendation may be most useful for patients who can benefit from short-term benzodiazepine treatment. Most guidelines suggest that benzodiazepine use should not exceed six weeks due to the potential for dependency. Further, benzodiazepines are associated with rebound anxiety, in which patients who have developed a tolerance become more anxious as they start to withdrawal. Finally, it may be difficult to determine the efficacy of an antidepressant due to the impact of benzodiazepine use. Due to the aforementioned factors, many psychopharmacological clinicians use benzodiazepines sparingly. Table 2 lists all of the currently available antidepressants and their FDA-approved as well as common off-label psychiatric uses.

Table 2. Commonly used antidepressants by class

Generic name	Trade name	FDA-approved psychiatric indications	Common off-label uses
Class: SSRI			
Fluoxetine	Prozac/Sarafem	MDD, OCD, PmDD, PTSD, PD, Bulimia	Anx, Soc Anx
Sertraline	Zoloft	MDD, OCD, PmDD, PTSD, PD, Soc Anx	Anx

(Continued)

Table 2. (*Continued*)

Generic name	Trade name	FDA-approved psychiatric indications	Common off-label uses
Paroxetine	Paxil/Pexeva	MDD, OCD, GAD, PD, Soc Anx, PTSD	Anx, PmDD
*Fluvoxamine		OCD	MDD, PTSD, Soc Anx, GAD
Citalopram	Celexa	MDD	Anx, PD, Soc Anx
Escitalorpam	Lexapro	MDD, GAD	Anx, PD, Soc Anx
Class: SNRI			
Venlafaxine	Effexor	MDD, GAD	PTSD, Anx Soc Anx
Duloxetine	Cymbalta	MDD	Anx
Class: SNRI (plus nonselective alpha 2 antagonism)			
Mirtazapine	Remeron	MDD	mild dep/low weight
Class: SARI			
*Nefazadone		MDD	Anx, PTSD, PD, GAD
Trazadone	Desyrel	MDD	Hyp
Class: Tricyclic			
Clomipramine	Anafranil	OCD	
Imipramine	Tofranil	MDD, enuresis	
Amitriptyline	Elavil	MDD	
Nortriptyline	Aventyl	MDD	
Maprotiline	Ludiomil	MDD	
Amoxapine	Asendin	MDD	
Doxepin	Sinequan/Adapin	MDD	
Trimipramine	Surmontil	MDD	
Desipramine	Norpramin	MDD	
Class: MAOI			
Tranylcypromine	Parnate	MDD	
Phenelzine	Nardil	MDD	
Isocarboxazid	Marplan	MDD	

Data from "Checklist and Uses of 100 Common Psychotropic Medications" by Dan Egli, PhD and Ed Zuckerman, PhD, 2005 (http://www.psychmeds.info/) and Essential Psychopharmacology: Neuroscientific Basis and Practical Applications by Stephen Stahl, MD, New York: Cambridge University Press, 2000. (78)

Abbreviations: MDD, major depressive disorder; OCD, obsessive compulsive disorder; PD, panic disorder; GAD, generalized anxiety disorder; PTSD, post-traumatic stress disorder; PmDD, premenstrual dysphoric disorder; Soc Anx, social anxiety disorder; mild dep/low weight, mild depressive symptoms in combination with difficulty gaining weight (usually in older adults)

*Available only in generic form

MEDICATIONS FOR ANXIETY DISORDERS

Not only is anxiety common in the general population, it is common among medical patients. Anxiety disorders are somewhat more difficult to diagnose because the different disorders can have overlapping symptoms as well as high comorbidity with MDD and other anxiety disorders. In fact, over 50 percent

as effective, if not more effective, than medications. So in cases in which a patient wishes to be referred to a mental health treatment provider, referring for psychotherapy can be a good first choice. Table 3 lists additional medications that are used in the treatment of anxiety disorders.

Table 3. Additional medications used in the treatment of anxiety

Generic name	Trade name	FDA-approved psychiatric Indications
Class: Serotonin 1A agonist		
Buspirone	Buspar	Anx
Class: Short-acting benzodiazepines		
Oxazepam	Serax	anx, etoh w/d
Alproazolam	Xanax	PD, anx
Triazolam	Halcion	shrt trm insom tx
Alprazolam	Niravam	PD, anx
Class: Mid-acting benzodiazepines		
Lorazepam	Ativan	anx, shrt trm insom tx
Estazolam	Prosam	shrt trm insom tx
Tamazepam	Restoril	shrt trm insom tx
Class: Long-acting benzodiazepines		
Clonazepam	Klonopin	PD, anx
Diazepam	Valium	anx, etoh w/d
Chlordiazepoxide	Librium	anx, etoh w/d
Flurazepam	Dalmane	shrt trm insom tx

Data from "Checklist and Uses of 100 common Psychotropic Medications" by Dan Egli, PhD and Ed Zuckerman, PhD, 2005 (http://www.psychmeds.info/) and Essential Psychopharmacology: Neuroscientific Basis and Practical Applications by Stephen Stahl, MD, New York: Cambridge University Press, 2000. (78)

Abbreviations: PD, panic disorder; anx, anxiety; shrt trm insom tx, short term insomnia treatment; etoh w/d, alcohol withdrawal

GENERALIZED ANXIETY DISORDER

Generalized anxiety disorder (GAD) is the most common anxiety disorder encountered in primary care.[17] GAD is characterized by excessive worry that is hard for the patient to control. Patients with GAD tend to describe themselves as "worriers," and asking patients if they would describe themselves this way is a key screening question. An answer of "yes" to whether a patient regards himself or herself as a worrier should prompt further interviewing for additional GAD criteria. Almost two-thirds of patients with GAD also have MDD.[26] Table 4 reviews the criteria for GAD as well as initial screening questions, which highlight the key diagnostic criteria for this disorder.

Newer generation antidepressants are frequently used in the treatment of GAD and research suggests that tricyclic antidepressants are also effective.[26] Some experts recommend the use of SSRIs as the first-line treatment for anxiety disorders.[27] Benzodiazepines are also effective in treating GAD, but concern about side effects and dependency often make their long-term use for treatment of anxiety disorders less desirable.[28-30]

Table 4. Diagnostic criteria for generalized anxiety disorder (GAD)

Excessive anxiety and worry occurring more days than not for at least six months

The worry is difficult to control

1. The anxiety and worry are associated with three or more of the following:
   Restlessness or feeling keyed up or edge
   Being easily fatigued
   Difficulty concentrating or mind going blank
   Irritability
   Muscle tension
   Sleep disturbance (difficulty initiating or maintaining sleep or restless sleep)
2. Anxiety is not due to worry about having a panic attack, fear of public embarrassment, or of being contaminated, which would indicate the presence of another anxiety disorder

Initial screening questions

1. Would you describe yourself as a worrier?
2. Do you find that once you are worrying about something that it is hard to stop the worry?

Reprinted with permission from the Diagnostic and Statistical Manual of Mental Disorders, Fourth Edition, Text Revision, (Copyright 2000). American Psychiatric Association.

Buspirone is also effective in the treatment of GAD, although it has no antidepressant effect.[27] Therefore, patients on buspirone should be thoroughly evaluated to ensure that they do not have comorbid depressive

PANIC DISORDER

Panic disorder is also common in medical patients, particularly those with cardiac disease and gastrointestinal problems or in about 4 percent of primary care patients.[31] Panic disorder involves the presence of recurrent, unexpected panic attacks. A panic attack is a discrete period in which the patient experiences intense anxiety involving both cognitive and somatic symptoms. Cognitive symptoms include fearfulness or terror, and somatic symptoms include shortness of breath, heart palpitations, chest pain, or choking sensations. Panic attacks occur with or without agoraphobia. Table 5 reviews criteria for panic disorder as well as initial screening questions.

Antidepressants are again commonly prescribed in the pharmacological treatment of panic disorder, with SSRIs and serotonin and noradrenaline reuptake inhibitors (SNRIs) often considered the first-line choice.[32] It has been documented that symptoms of panic disorder can worsen initially in treatment with antidepressants. This "onset worsening" is not seen with other anxiety disorders or in the treatment of depression.[27] TCAs are also an option for treatment, as is acute dosing with benzodiazepines, preferably those with longer half-lives to avoid rebound anxiety.[29]

POST-TRAUMATIC STRESS DISORDER

As discussed in Chapter 4, post-traumatic stress disorder symptoms are common in medical populations. Some studies suggest that as many as 30 percent of cancer patients develop PTSD and 29 percent of coronary heart disease patients also develop the disorder.[33,34]

Table 5. Diagnostic criteria for panic disorder (PD)

Criteria for a panic attack

1. A discrete period of intense fear and discomfort, in which four or more of the following develop abruptly and reach a peak within ten minutes:
   Palpitations, pounding heart or accelerated heart rate
   Sweating
   Trembling or shaking
   Sensation of shortness of breath or choking
   Chest pain or discomfort
   Nausea or abdominal distress
   Feeling dizzy, light-headed, or faint
   Derealization (feeling of unreality) or depersonalization (feeling detatched from oneself)
   Fear of losing control or going crazy
   Fear of dying
   Paresthesias
   Chills or hot flushes
2. There must be at least one month of persistent concern about having another panic attack, worry about the consequences of panic attacks, or behavioral change related to the attacks

Criteria for agoraphobia:

1. Anxiety about being in places in which escape might be difficult in the event of a panic attack, including being outside of the home alone, crowded places, standing in line, being on bridges, etc.
2. These situations are avoided or are endured with marked distress and anxiety about having a panic attack

Initial screening questions

1. Do you ever have times where you find yourself suddenly anxious and overwhelmed?
2. Does this anxiety get very intense within 10–15 minutes?
3. Do you have physical symptoms with this anxiety?

Reprinted with permission from the Diagnostic and Statistical Manual of Mental Disorders, Fourth Edition, Text Revision, (Copyright 2000). American Psychiatric Association.

Table 6 reviews the criteria for PTSD and provides initial screening questions. Research on the pharmacology of PTSD is plagued by the same difficulties as research on the prevalence of PTSD; it is difficult to study because of the wide range of traumatic events that can cause PTSD symptoms and the diverse presentations in patients. As a result, there has been relatively little research on pharmacology in this patient population, and much of the research that exists involves small sample sizes and lacks control group comparisons. Nevertheless, antidepressants are widely

Table 6. Diagnostic criteria for post-traumatic stress disorder (PTSD)

1. The person experienced, witnessed, or was confronted with a traumatic event that involved actual or threatened death or a threat to the physical integrity of self or others and the person's response to the event was intense fear, helpless

   Withdrawal from others
   Emotional numbing
   Sense of a foreshortened future
4. Two or more symptoms of increased arousal:
   Insomnia
   Irritability
   Concentration difficulties
   Hypervigilance
   Exaggerated startle response

   Initial screening questions
   1. Have you ever experienced anything that you consider traumatic?
   2. Do you find that you think about this experience, even when you don't want to or have dreams about it?

Reprinted with permission from the Diagnostic and Statistical Manual of Mental Disorders, Fourth Edition, Text Revision, (Copyright 2000). American Psychiatric Association.

prescribed for PTSD. Though there is no evidence that any one particular class of medications is more useful than another in symptom reduction, much of the research has been with serotonergic agents, and it has been hypothesized that these agents may be more efficacious than TCAs.[35] The efficacy of MAOIs has had mixed findings in PTSD populations.[36] Other agents suggested in the literature include low-dose, atypical antipsychotics as well as anticonvulsants such as lamotrigine, gabapentin, carbamazepine, and valproic acid. However, the research on these agents has been limited, and sample sizes that have examined these agents have been small.[17,36] Given the limited research on medications in this population as well as the complicated psychosocial aspects of these patients, many experts recommend a first trial of psychotherapy before initiating drug treatment, depending on symptom severity.

DRUG INTERACTIONS AND SPECIAL CONSIDERATIONS IN MEDICAL AND GERIATRIC PATIENTS

In recent years a wide range of psychotropic drugs has become available, but some of these drugs should be used cautiously in patients taking multiple medications or in older adults whose have decreased metabolic functioning. Many interactions concerning psychiatric drugs involve the cytochrome P450 (CYP 450) system in the liver, as many of these drugs inhibit or induce liver isoenzymes. Induction or inhibition can impact the metabolism of psychotropic as well as other types of medications, although not all of these interactions are clinically significant. In fact, while many drugs can and do interact with one another, in most cases these interactions appear not to be clinically significant, although research is continuing to investigate this. In cases in which medication interactions are significant, however, induction or inhibition of CYP 450 enzymes can decrease or increase levels of the inducer or inhibitor or the medication impacted by the alteration in metabolism (substrate). Enzyme inhibition, however, is usually associated with more severe drug interactions. This section will identify some common medication combinations involving antidepressants and benzodiazepines that can produce more severe drug interactions, as well as medications that are a relatively lower risk for drug interactions. Table 7 lists antidepressant medications that are CYP 450 inhibitors.

All SSRIs interact with the CYP 450 system. Some SSRIs, as well as other classes of antidepressants, inhibit the CYP enzyme 2D6, which is an important enzyme in some drug interactions. Additionally, genetic polymorphisms exist among 2D6, and 5 percent to 10 percent of Caucasians and 18 percent of West Africans are poor metabolizers of 2D6, meaning that these individuals may be at risk of drug interactions with medications inhibiting this enzyme.[37] The most potent inhibitors of this enzyme are bupropion, paroxetine, and fluoxetine.[38] In addition to being a potent inhibitor of CYP2D6, fluoxetine also has a long half-life and an active metabolite, norfluoxetine. Fluoxetine's long half-life is often considered beneficial for patients who may not be consistent in taking their antidepressant, but it can be problematic when it is co-administered with other medications because stopping the medication if necessary will not stop medication interactions potentially for several weeks. Additionally, after stopping fluoxetine, great caution is advised in adding a serotonergic agent

Table 7. Antidepressants that act as inhibitors in CYP 450-mediated drug interactions

	Level of		Level of
sertraline	+	venlafaxine	+
2C19 inhibitors		2C9 inhibitors	
fluoxetine	++	fluvoxamine	+
fluvoxamine	+++	paroxetine	++
paroxetine	+++	sertraline	+++
1A2			
fluvoxamine	+		

+, mild inhibition; ++, moderate inhibition; +++, potent inhibition
Note: Data from references 37, 38, 40, and 55

because of the risk of serotonin syndrome (which will be described in more detail in the next section). Studies have found that the inhibition of 2D6 by fluoxetine has impacted the clearance of desipramine, thus increasing desipramine levels without a change in dose.[39] A recent review of drug interactions concerning antidepressants cited that fluoxetine may cause a twofold to fourfold increase in plasma concentrations for all of the TCAs and that a similar increase in TCA levels has been reported in patients taking paroxetine.[40] Fluoxetine also impacts the clearance of alprazolam. Several studies have demonstrated that fluoxetine can decrease the clearance of alprazolam, resulting in reduced psychomotor performance and impaired short-term memory.[41] Thus, dosing of alprazolam should be reduced when co-administering with fluoxetine. Fluoxetine can also increase the plasma concentration of traditional antipsychotics such as halperidol and fluphenazine as well as some of the atypical antipsychotics, including clozapine and resperidone.[40]

Inhibitors of CYP 2D6 have been thought to interfere with the metabolism of drugs that convert to morphine, such as codeine, although some researchers do not agree that codeine relies on 2D6 for conversion to morphine and this issue is still being investigated.[42] If it is the case that codeine relies on 2D6 to convert to morphine, then it is possible that persons who receive medications that are potent inhibitors of this enzyme may have reduced analgesia. This has been speculated in the literature.[42,43] In my experience, I have seen patients who have been on fluoxetine and morphine report better pain control when switched to antidepressants such as mirtazapine or citalopram. Although the research may be unclear as to whether these medications constitute a true and significant interaction, many patients can be viewed as medication-seeking if they complain of inadequate analgesia. Given the possible interactions of codeine and morphine derivatives and medications that inhibit 2D6, it may be prudent to try another antidepressant to see if analgesia is improved. This may help to rule out medication seeking or inadequate pain control that is due to other factors.

Among the SSRIs, those that have relatively low profiles for drug interactions, as documented in the literature to date, are sertraline, citalopram, and escitalopram.[44–47] One caveat, however, regarding sertraline is that this medication (as well as fluoxetine and fluvoxamine) is an inhibitor of CYP 3A4. Therefore, it should not be co-administered with astemizole due to the possibility of lethal arrythmias.[48] Additionally, citalopram is potentially problematic for patients taking warfarin, as discussed below. Among the newer antidepressants, venlafaxine and mirtazapine have relatively low potential for interactions. Since nefazadone is a potent inhibitor of CYP 3A4, it has been shown to increase plasma levels of carbamazepine and haloperidol.[40] This same review article reported that nefazadone should not be given with astemizole or loratadine due to a predisposition of the fatal ventricular dysrhythmia torsades de pointes.

Inhibitors of 2C19 are fluvoxamine, fluoxetine, and paroxetine.[40] Although there have not been a number of clinically significant drug interactions reported with 2C19 inhibitors and substrates, it is important to note that significant polymorphism exists for this isoenzyme. From 18 percent to 23 percent of Japanese nationals have been found lack the 2C19 isoenzyme as well as up to 20 percent of persons in other Asian populations.[49,50] Therefore, careful monitoring for adverse effects is warranted in administering 2C19 inhibitors in these populations.

As the reader likely knows, warfarin interacts with multiple medications. Among the antidepressants, it is probable that citalopram, sertraline, and fluvoxamine potentiate warfarin and that trazadone inhibits it.[51] Additionally, other research cautions against the use of fluoxetine with warfarin because it inhibits CYP3A4 and could be associated with excessive

populations in which anticholinergic effects can lead to constipation, urinary retention, and memory impairment.

St. John's wort is a popular herbal medication that is used in the treatment of depression. Although in current practice physicians routinely ask patients what herbal medications they are taking, in medically complicated patients information on herbal supplements may be left out in history taking. St. John's wort has been increasingly recognized as potentially problematic when co-administered with other drugs. In general, it is recommended to avoid St. John's wort or to use it with extreme caution in patients who are taking agents that act on serotonin, norepinephrine, or dopamine due to the risk of serotonin syndrome.[56] St. John's wort is a potent inducer of CYP 3A4. A recent review article reported that St. John's wort decreased the concentration of a number of drugs including amitriptyline, cyclosporine, digoxin, fexofenadine, indinavir, methadone, midazolam, nevirapine, phenprocoumon, simvastatin, tacrolimus, theophylline, and warfarin.[57] This review also reported, consistent with multiple case reports of women of child-bearing age, that using St. John's wort with oral contraceptives can lead to breakthrough bleeding and unplanned pregnancies.

Medically ill and geriatric patients are at risk for drug interactions because of the impact of aging on metabolism as well as the effects of multiple medications. Many medication interactions are possible. This section has only briefly addressed some of the possible interactions among antidepressants and other medications and has been limited to metabolic interactions commonly described in the literature. As research in this area is ongoing, it is likely that other interactions will be discovered. Table 8 lists resources where clinicians can find more information on psychiatric medications and drug–drug interactions.

Table 8. Additional resources regarding psychiatric medications and drug–drug interactions

Websites

Basic psychopharmacology information and drug tables:
www.psychmeds.info/
Information regarding drug interactions:
http://mhc.com/Cytochromes/
http://www.drug-interactions.com
http://www.preskorn.com
Manual for the Texas Medication Algorithm:
http://www.dshs.state.tx.us/mhprograms/TMAPover.shtm

Books

Pharmacology and psychopharmacology:
Basic and Clinical Pharmacology, Katzung, BG, editor: Lange Medical Books/McGraw Hill: 2003
Essential Psychopharmacology (Essential Psychopharmacology Series) Stahl, SM. Cambridge University Press: 2000
Essential Psychopharmacology: The Prescriber's Guide (Essential Psychopharmacology Series) Stahl, SM. Cambridge University Press: 2005

A good general rule with medical patients is to consider the potential impact of adding an antidepressant or anxiolytic and to remember that an addition of medication in this population may not be benign. Thus, the "Start Low and Go Slow" strategy is wise.[58] In observing this principle, I often suggest starting geriatric or medically ill patients on half of the recommended starting dose of an antidepressant and evaluating tolerance before increasing to the recommended starting dose. This strategy not only seems to minimize side effects, but also allows clinicians to monitor for drug interactions. It should be noted that in this model I or another clinician have frequent contact with the patient to monitor mood symptoms and adverse effects.

SCREENING FOR ALCOHOL AND CAFFEINE USE

Alcohol and caffeine are the two most widely used controlled substances in the world.[59] Because of the wide use of these substances and their psychoactive effects, clinicians should screen for use of these substances prior to prescribing psychotropic medications.

Primary care clinicians provide care for a number of patients with alcohol problems and prevalence rates of alcohol abuse and dependency in primary care patients range from 2 to 29 percent.[60] Alcohol is a central nervous sys-

or her alcohol use, if others are bothered by the patient's drinking, whether he or she experiences guilt related to drinking, and if they have alcohol upon awakening are questions that are sensitive in detecting an alcohol problem.

Caffeine, which is used even more widely than alcohol, is a powerful central nervous system stimulant. It is present in coffee, tea, colas, and chocolate. Most of us are well aware of its rewarding effects on alertness and energy level. Since caffeine is a stimulant, it poses problems for patients with anxiety. Anxious patients who use caffeine tend to have more anxiety. Additionally, sensitivity to caffeine can last from eight to fourteen hours, thus significantly disrupting sleep for many people.[62] Screening for caffeine use in patients with anxiety is important because if patients are willing to cut down on caffeine use, anxiety may be able to be managed without the use of medications. Additionally, caffeine is metabolized CYP450 1A2, which can cause drug interactions with other 1A2 substrates. Fluvoxamine is also a substrate of 1A2.[63,64] Therefore, screening patients who take fluvoxamine regarding caffeine use could help avoid a clinically significant drug interaction.

SPECIAL ISSUES IN THE USE OF SEROTONIN AGENTS

Although SSRIs and serotonergic agents are commonly and safely used throughout the world, there are a number of issues with these medications that are helpful to be aware of. These issues include serotonin syndrome, the warnings regarding suicidality, discontinuation syndrome, and sexual side effects.

Serotonin syndrome is a potentially life threatening reaction resulting from excessive serotonergic agonism and can occur not just with SSRIs, but any agent that acts on serotonin. Mild cases of serotonin syndrome can involve symptoms of tachycardia, shivering, akathisia, diaphoresis, myodriasis, tremor, myoclonus, and hyperreflexia. More severe symptoms include hypertension, hyperactive bowel sounds (and possibly diarrhea) hyperthermia, fever, diaphoresis, sustained clonus, altered mental status, and shock.[65] Milder cases of serotonin syndrome can be misperceived as anxiety because akathisia is generally characterized by motor restlessness, which can also be a symptom of anxiety. In contrast to anxiety, however, akathisia often involves a feeling muscular quivering and patients describe that they feel as if they want to "jump out of their skin." Any increase in anxiety or psychomotor agitation should prompt further investigation to rule out serotonin syndrome. Management of serotonin syndrome involves stopping the precipitating drug and supportive care.

In 2003 the Medicine and Health care Products Regulatory Agency of the British Department of Health warned physicians to avoid the off-label use of paroxetine for the treatment of children with depression.[66] The report of an increase in suicidal behavior in children on antidepressants has since received world wide attention as well as speculation regarding what these findings might mean for adults. (The issues associated with the use of antidepressants in children involve a number of risk/benefit related concerns and are beyond the scope of this chapter. The interested reader should refer to the medical literature and FDA data on efficacy and risks of the use of antidepressants in children.) In the United States, the FDA issued a public health advisory regarding the use of antidepressants in adults. This advisory warns that patients who are started on antidepressants should be monitored for worsening depression, an increase in suicidal thinking or behavior, and that a worsening of these symptoms warrants further evaluation by a health care professional.[67] The issue of whether or not antidepressants increase the likelihood of suicidality is not without controversy. Many epidemiological studies in several European countries have found that in adults, antidepressant use decreases rates of suicidality and that many of these decreases coincided with the introduction of SSRIs.[68] In fact, these authors also conducted a longitudinal study on 521 patients on SSRIs and found a fourfold increase in suicidality when patients were off of SSRIs. Another review found that there is not consistent data to support the view that antidepressants worsen the course of depression, and other research continues to find that antidepressants reduce the risk of suicide.[69,70] Despite these findings and opinions, other researchers stand by the idea that adult patients taking SSRIs are twice as likely to attempt suicide as those taking a placebo. A review of the literature in the *British Medical Journal* found a more than twofold increase in sui-

and complicated. Nevertheless, the risk of suicide in depressed patients is, of course, a possible outcome. Depressed patients who are not on medication are also at risk of suicide. This fact reinforces the need to thoroughly screen patients for suicidal thinking and behaviors, the provision of frequent follow-up with patients following the initiation of an serotonergic agent, as well as the importance of referring to mental health professionals when necessary.

Discontinuation syndrome is another issue to be aware of with serotonergic agents. It has been described as involving five core somatic sets of symptoms:[73,74]

- Disequilibrium (dizziness, vertigo, ataxia)
- Gastrointestinal symptoms (nausea, vomiting, diarrhea)
- Flu-like symptoms (fatigue, lethargy, myalgia, chills)
- Sensory disturbances (shock-like paresthesia)
- Sleep disturbances (insomnia, vivid dreams)

As mentioned previously, paroxetine has the worst record for discontinuation syndrome (shock like paresthesia has also been reported in a small number of patients initiating paroxetine[74]) and fluoxetine has minimal withdrawal syndrome because of its long half-life. Therefore, standard recommendations are to slowly taper off of all serotonergic agents to minimize discontinuation symptoms.

All medications have the risk of long-term adverse effects and SSRIs and serotonin agents are no exception. Although many of the side effects with SSRIs are transient some persist well into treatment. Monitoring for side effects can help to prevent discontinuation and can help to address important issues related to quality of life.

Perhaps one of the most publicized side effects of SSRIs is sexual side effects. Sexual side effects associated with these medications include inhibition of libido, ejaculation, and orgasm. The range of reported sexual dysfunction ranges from 24 percent to 65 percent, depending on the study.[55,75,76] Bupriprion, nefazadone, and mirtazepine have been suggested as alternative medications for patients who develop sexual dysfunction.[55]

Overall, serotonin agents are safe and effective treatments for depression and a number of anxiety disorders. However, no medication is without risk. Perhaps because of the relatively low risk of newer antidepressants, these agents may have become overly prescribed or prescribed without frequent follow-up. The recent media attention given to the range of possible adverse effects of these medications serves as a reminder that, like all medications, antidepressants have the potential for serious consequences. However, with close follow-up and monitoring of patients, adverse events can be minimized.

CONCLUSIONS

Primary care physicians are major providers of mental health services in the United States and prescribe the majority of antidepressants that patients receive. Research suggests that although primary care clinicians are more than equipped to manage many mental health disorders, more follow-up is needed with patients once psychotropic medications are prescribed. Given the time constraints of many physicians, this is difficult, and many physicians resolve this issue by both prescribing an antidepressant and referring a patient for psychotherapy. Psychotherapists with proper training can monitor patients for adverse effects of medications, monitor mood symptoms, and can collaborate with physicians when dosage adjustments are needed or when adverse events occur. It is also important to remember that the expertise of a psychiatrist can be invaluable when patients have complicated psychiatric histories as well as difficulty tolerating initial trials of psychotropic medications. Collaboration with mental health professionals can not only ease the burden of primary care physicians, but improved patient outcomes have been found when general practitioners collaborate with psychologists or psychiatrists.[77] The decision whether to refer to a psychotherapist or to manage a patient's care independently depends on patient's preferences and physician comfort with the management of psychiatric disorders, as well as availability for follow-up. Chapter 9 will discuss the issues to consider when referring to a mental health clinician.

... p........./ ...... p...........,

3. Depression guideline panel. *Depression in Primary Care. Clinical Practice Guideline, No. 5*. Vol 2. Rockville, MD: Agency for Health Care Policy and Research; April 1993.

4. Mojitabai R. Diagnosing depression and prescribing antidepressants by primary care physicians: the impact of practice style variations. *Ment Health Serv Res.* 2002;4:109–118.

5. Weilburg JB, O'Leary KM, Meigs JB, Hennen J, Stafford RS. Evaluation of the adequacy of outpatient antidepressant treatment. *Psychiatr Serv.* 2003;54: 1233–1239.

6. Wilson I, Duszynski K, Mant A. A 5-year follow-up of general practice patients experiencing depression. *Fam. Pract.* 2003;20:685–689.

7. Bull SA, Hu XH, Hunkeler EM, et al. Discontinuation of use and switching of antidepressants: influence of patient–physician communication. *J Am Med Assoc.* 2002;288:1403–1409.

8. Nierenberg AA Wright EC. Evolution of remission as the new standard in the treatment of depression. *J Clin Psychiatry.* 1999;60(suppl 22):7–11.

9. Frank E, Karp JF, Rush AJ. Efficacy of treatments for major depression. *Psychopharmacol Bull.* 1993;29:457–475.

10. AHCPR. *Clinical practice guideline number 5: depression in primary care: treatment of major depression.* Vol 2. Rockville, MD: United States Department of Health and Human Services, Agency for Health care Policy and Research; 1993 [AHCPR publication 93-0551].

11. Thase ME, Sullivan LR. Relapse and recurrence of depression: a practical approach for prevention. *CNS Drugs.* 1995;4:261–277.

12. Sammons M. Introduction: the politics and pragmatics of prescriptive authority. In: Sammons M, Levant RF, Paige RU, eds. *Prescriptive Authority for Psychologists: a History and Guide.* Washington, DC: American Psychological Association; 2003:3–31.

13. Pettit JW, Voelz ZR, Joiner TE. Combined treatments for depression. In: Sammons M, Schmidt NB, eds. *Combined Treatments for Medical Disorders.* Washington, DC: American Psychological Association; 2001:131–159.

14. Nemeroff CB, Heim C, Thase ME, et al. Differential responses to psychotherapy versus pharmacotherapy in patients with chronic forms of major depression and childhood trauma. *Proc Natl Acad Sci USA.* 2003;25:14293–14296 [E pub].

15. APA. *Diagnostic and Statistical Manual of Mental Disorders.* 4th ed., text rev. Washington, DC: American Psychiatric Association; 2000.

16. Whooley MA. Simon GE. Managing depression in medical outpatients. *N Engl J Med.* 2000;343:1942–1950.

17. Kjernisted KD. Long-term goals in the management of acute and chronic anxiety disorders. *Can J Psychiatry.* 2004;49(suppl 1):51S–63S.

18. Perlis RH, Fraguas R, Fava M, et al. Prevalence and clinical correlates of irritability in major depressive disorder: a preliminary report from the sequenced treatment alternatives to relieve depression study. *J Clin Psychiatry.* 2005;66: 159–166.

19. Mulrow CD, Williams Jr JW, Chiquette E, et al. Efficacy of newer medications for treating depression in primary care patients. *Am J Med.* 2000;108:54–64.

20. Trivedi MH, Rush AJ, Crismon ML, et al. Clinical results for patients with major depressive disorder in the Texas medication algorithm project. *Arch Gen Psychiatry.* 2004;61:669–680.

21. Lam R, Kennedy SH. Evidence-based strategies for achieving and sustaining full remission in depression: focus on metaanalyses. *Can J Psychiatry.* 2004;49 (suppl 1):17S–26S.

22. Stahl SM. *Essential Psychopharmacology of Depression and Bipolar Disorder.* Cambridge: Cambridge University; 2000.

23. Green B. Focus on paroxetine. *Curr Med Res Opin.* 2003;19:13–21.

24. Furukawa TA, Streiner DL, Young LT. Antidepressants and benzodiazepine for major depression. *Cochrane Database Syst Rev.* 2001 [Art. No.: CD001026. DOI:10.1002/14651858.CD001026].

25. Culpepper L. Use of algorithms to treat anxiety in primary care. *J Clin Psychiatry.* 2003;64(suppl 2):30–33.

26. Kapczinski F, Lima MS, Souza JS, Schmitt R. Antidepressants for generalized anxiety disorder. *Cochrane Database Syst Rev.* 2003 [Art. No.: CD003592, DOI:10.1002/14651858.CD003592].

27. Ballenger JC, Davidson JRT, Lecrubier Y, Nutt DJ. A proposed algorithm for improved recognition and treatment of the depression/anxiety spectrum in primary care. *Prim Care Companion J Clin Psychiatry.* 2001;3:44–52.

28. Fricchione G. Generalized anxiety disorder. *N Engl J Med.* 2004;351:675–682.

29. Stein DJ. Algorithms for primary care: an evidence-based approach to the pharmacology of depression and anxiety disorders. *Prim Psychiatry.* 2004;11:55–78.

30. Gorman JM. Treating generalized anxiety disorder. *J Clin Psychiatry.* 2003;64(suppl 2):24–29.

31. Roy-Byrne PP, Wagner AW, Schraufnagel BS. Understanding and treating panic disorder in the primary care setting. *J Clin Psychiatry.* 2005;66(suppl 4):16–22.

32. Pollack MH. The pharmacotherapy of panic disorder. *J Clin Psychiatry.* 2005;66(suppl 4):23–27.

33. Kangas M, Henry JL, Bryant RA. Posttraumatic stress disorder following

cal review. *J Psychiatr Res.* 2002;36:355–367.

37. Bernard SA, Brera E. Drug interactions in palliative care. *J Clin Oncol.* 2000;18:1780–1799.

38. Preskorn SH, Flockhart D. Guide to psychiatric drug interactions. *Prim Psychiatry.* 2004;11:39–60.

39. Preskorn SH, Aldereman J, Chung M, et al. Pharmacokinetics of desipramine co-administered with sertraline or fluoxetine. *J Clin Psychopharmacol.* 1994;2: 90–98.

40. Spina E, Scordo MG, D'Arrigo C. Metabolic drug interactions with new psychotropic agents. *Fundam Clin Pharmacol.* 2003;17:517–38.

41. Chouinard G, Lefko-Singh K, Teboul E. Metabolism of anxiolytics and hypnotics: benzodiazepines, buspirone, zoplicone, and zolpidem. *Cell Mol Neurobiol.* 1999;19:533–552.

42. Armstrong SC, Cozza KL. Pharmacokinetic drug interactions of morphine, codeine, and their derivatives: theory and clinical reality, part II. *Psychosomatics.* 2003;44:515–520.

43. Preskorn SH. Multiple medications, multiple considerations. *J Psychiat Pract.* 2001;48–52. http://www.pre3swkorn.com/columns/0101.html; Accessed 07.10.05.

44. Muijsers RB, Plosker GL, Noble S. Sertraline: a review of its use in the management of major depressive disoder in elderly patients. *Drugs Aging.* 2002;19:377–392.

45. Brosen K, Naranjo CA. Review of pharmacokinetic and pharmacodynamic interaction studies with citalopram. *Eur Neuropsychopharmacol.* 2001; 11:275–283.

46. Malin P, Wengel SP, Burke WJ. Escitalopram: better treatment for depression is through the looking glass. *Expert Rev Neurother.* 2004;4:769–779.

47. Crone CC, Gabriel GM. Treatment of anxiety and depression in transplant patients: pharmacokinetic considerations. *Clin Pharmacokinet.* 2004;43:361–94.

48. Mulchahey JJ, Malik MS, Sabai M, Kasckow JW. Serotonin-selective reuptake inhibitors in the treatment of geriatric depression and related disorders. *Int J Neuropsychopharmacol.* 1999;2:121–127.

49. Flockhart D. Drug interactions and the cytochrome P450 system: the role of P450 2C19. *Clin Pharmacokinet.* 1995;29:45–52.

50. Ereshefsky L. Treating depression: potential drug–drug interactions. *J Clin Psychopharmacol.* 1996;16:50S–53S.

51. Holbrook AM, Pereira JA, Labiris R, et al. Systematic overview of warfarin and its drug and food interactions. *Arch Int Med* 2005;165:1095–1106.

52. Johnson MD, Newkirk G, White JR. *Clinically Significant Drug Interactions*; 1999 [Post Grad Med 1999; 105]. http://www.postgradmed.com/issues/1999/0299/johnson.htm; Accessed.

53. Hyttel J. Pharmacological characterization of selective serotonin reuptake inhibitors (SSRIs). *Int Clin Psychopharmacol.* 1994;9(suppl 1):19–26.

54. Fujishiro J, Taiichiro I, Onozawa K, Tsushima M. Comparison of the anticholinergic effects of the serotonergic antidepressants, paroxetine, fluvoxamine and clomipramine. *Eur J Pharmacol.* 2002;454:183–188.

55. Masand PS, Gupta S. Long-term side effects of newer generation antidepressants: SSRIs, venlafaxine, nefazodone, bupropion, and mirtazapine. *Ann Clin Psychiatry.* 2002;143:175–182.

56. Dennehy CE, Tsourounis C. Botanical ("herbal medications") & nutritional supplements. In: Katzung BG, ed. *Basic and Clinical Pharmacology.* New York: Lange Medical Books/McGraw-Hill;2001:1088–1103.

57. Zhou S, Chan E, Pan SQ, Huang M, Lee EJ. Pharmacokinetic interactions of drugs with St. John's wort. *J Psychopharmacol.* 2004;18:262–276.

58. Young RC, Meyers BS. Psychophramacology. In: Sadovoy J, Lazarus LW, Jarvik LF, et al., eds. *Comprehensive Review of Geriatric Psychiatry II.* Washington, DC: American Psychiatric Press; 1996:755–817.

59. Julien RM. *A Primer of Drug Action.* New York: Worth Publishers; 2001.

60. Fiellin DA, Reid C, O'Connor PG. Screening for alcohol problems in primary care. *Arch Int Med.* 2000;160:1977–1989.

61. Mayfield D, McLeod G, Hall P. The CAGE questionnaire: validation of a new alcoholism screening instrument. *Am J Psychiatry.* 1974;131:1121–1123.

62. Zarcone VP. Sleep hygiene. In: Kryger MH, Roth T, Dement WC, eds. *Principals and Practice of Sleep Medicine.* 3rd ed. Philadelphia: W.B. Saunders Company; 2000:657–661.

63. Carrillo JA, Dahl ML, Svensson JO, et al. Disposition of fluvoxamine in humans is determined by the polymorphic CYP2D6 and also by the CYP1A2 activity. *Clin Pharmacol Ther.* 1996;60:183–190.

64. Carrillo JA, Benitez J. Clinically significant pharmacokinetic interactions between dietary caffeine and medications. *Clin Pharmacokinet.* 2000;39:127–153.

65. Boyer EW, Shannon M. The serotonin syndrome. *N Engl J Med.* 2005;352:1112–1120.

66. Vitiello B, Swedo S. Antidepressant medications in children. *N Engl J Med.* 2004;350:1489–1491.

67. *FDA public health advisory: suicidality in adults being treated with antidepressant medications.* http://www.fda.gov/cder/drug/advisory/SSRI200507.htm; Accessed 23.12.05.

71. Fergusson D, Doucette S, Glass KC, et al. Association between suicide attempts and selective serotonin reuptake inhibitors: Systematic review of randomized controlled clinical trials. *BMJ.* 2005;330:396.
72. Lenzer J. FDA warns that antidepressants may increase suicidality in adults. *BMJ.* 2005;331:70.
73. Zajecka J, Tracy KA, Mitchell S. Serotonin reuptake inhibitor discontinuation syndrome: a hypothetical definition. *J Clin Psychiatry.* 1997;58:291–297.
74. Berigan TR, Cannard AW, Cannard KR. Transient paroxysmal, shock-like paresthesias associated with paroxetine initiation. *J Clin Psychiatry.* 1997;58:175–76.
75. Hu XH, Bull SA, Hunkeler EM, et al. Incidence and duration of side effects and those rated as bothersome with selective serotonin reuptake inhibitor treatment for depression: Patient report versus physician estimate. *J Clin Psychiatry.* 2004;65:959–965.
76. Landén M, Högberg B, Thase ME. Incidence of sexual side effects in refractory depression during treatment with citalopram or paroxetine. *J Clin Psychiatry* 2005;66:100–106.
77. Schulberg HC, Katon W, Simon GE, Rush AJ. Treating major depression in primary care practice. *Arch Gen Psychiatry.* 1998;55:1121–1127.
78. Stahl SM. *Essential Psychopharmacology: Neuroscientific Basis and Practical Applications.* New York: Cambridge University Press; 2000.

6

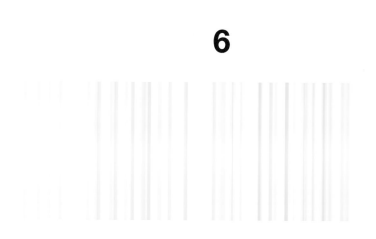

"A man's illness is his private territory, and, no matter how much he loves you and how close you are, you stay an outsider. You are healthy."
—Lauren Bacall

Family members, spouses and partners, and friends of patients are obviously impacted by a patient's illness. While these important persons spend far more time with patients than either physicians or the mental health professionals who provide care, family members are frequently, albeit unintentionally, left out as important players in the care and management of persons who are chronically ill. There are likely many reasons for this. First, busy physicians may not feel they have the time to devote to family members. Especially for patients that are seriously ill, conversations with family members can be long and involved. Second, some family members may feel intimidated by physicians or see physicians as the ultimate authority. This is especially true among elderly persons or persons from cultures in which authority is given high respect. In such cases, family members may feel uncomfortable with asking a physician questions or taking an active role in the patient's care. Additionally, many family members are aware of the needs of the patient and seem intentionally to keep a low profile when around physicians so as not to interfere with their loved one's care. Third, in some instances, physicians are under intense pressure to provide concrete answers to family members regarding a patient's condition and prognosis. In some cases, often involving very sick patients, physicians cannot provide definite answers regarding the prognosis and avoid having discussions with family members as a result. For example, one physician, who had several very sick ventilated patients, told me that he goes to the facility to see his patients when family members are not likely to be around to avoid difficult conversations in which he cannot provide answers. Fourth, family dynamics can be extremely complicated. When family dynamics are tense or hostile, physicians often want to avoid being in the middle of conflict or being targeted by angry family members. Consider the following case example:

> Kathy is a 55-year-old woman with a long history of medical illness, including coronary heart failure (CHF), peripheral vascular disease, depression, and chronic back pain secondary to two motor vehicle accidents over twenty-years ago. She was admitted to the hospital for a CHF exacerbation. While hospitalized, she developed a nosocomial line infection, which prolonged her stay due to need of intravenous antibiotics. Kathy lived with her 33-year-old son Rob, who was her primary caretaker. During the hospital stay, staff noticed that Rob and Kathy would argue vehemently. Different staff had different perspectives on these arguments. Some staff felt that Kathy was mistreating her son and had unrealistic expectations of him. Others felt that Rob was verbally abusive to his mother and that he was financially exploiting her, and they wondered if a report should be made to Adult Protective Services. The reality of this situation was probably somewhere between these two perceptions. Rob became fiercely protective of his mother, and this protectiveness manifested itself as anger when physicians came to see Kathy. He accused them of providing poor care, of intentionally prolonging her stay so that the hospital could earn more money, and of not having a plan for her discharge. Kathy said nothing during these outbursts, but the physicians who attempted to talk to Kathy about her treatment as well as discharge plans felt helpless and insulted. Not surprisingly, they avoided Kathy and her son, allowing nursing staff to communicate to them about Kathy's status and needs. As a result, Kathy's discharge was delayed due to lack of communication among physicians treating Kathy as well as with administrators who were in charge of arranging discharge.

When patients get sick, family members are an intimate part of the illness. The illness also occurs in the context of family emotional problems. As with intrapsychic issues, illness doesn't make the problems that existed

When families feel left out of patient care, this can lead to later problems, especially as illness progresses. Since there has been relatively little discussion of dealing with family members in the literature, I will focus more on problematic aspects of dealing with families and will present some guidelines that may help physicians deal with family members in difficult situations.

CAREGIVER STRESS, GUILT, AND ANXIETY

Approximately 25 percent of the U.S. population reports that they provide care to a family member or friend with chronic or terminal illness.[1] The psychological impact of caring for a loved one who is ill is significant. One study interviewed two hundred caretakers of advanced cancer patients and found that 13 percent of these caretakers met criteria for a psychiatric disorder using *Diagnostic and Statistical Manual of Mental Disorders* criteria.[2] The disorders in this population included depression, post-traumatic stress disorder, and generalized anxiety disorder. Other research has found that caregivers report lower physical and psychological well-being than noncaregivers, but this result is more robust in persons caring for patients with dementia.[3,4] This finding is also stronger in ethnic minorities, with Asian and Hispanic caretakers reporting more depression than white and African-American caretakers.[4]

The issues affecting family members of ill patients are multiple. When patients are caring for a family member in their home, in a hospital, or in a nursing facility, family members sometimes feel as if they always have to be available for the patient. Consider the situation of Sharon:

Sharon was a 56-year-old woman referred by her primary care physician for psychotherapy related to the stress of taking care of her mother. Her mother was 86-years-old and lived in a highly reputed facility that specialized in taking care of patients with Alzheimer's dementia. Sharon reported that she and her mother never had a good relationship and openly acknowledged that she felt resentful of her mother. Sharon was the youngest of four children and felt that her mother had spent little time with her and had been preoccupied with her other children. Sharon also felt that her father was inattentive to her mother and reported that her father had multiple extramarital relationships. Yet, though Sharon's other siblings were reportedly closer to her mother, Sharon was the main person in the family providing care for her mother. She had Deputy Power of Attorney and made all health care decisions. Sharon frequently reported that she was overwhelmed by her mother's needs and that though multiple staff members attended to her mother's care, she felt the care was inadequate. She had stopped working and visited her mother almost every day and had frequent arguments with staff regarding the quality of care. She also became very angry with the physician who was taking care of her mother and accused him of not attending to her mother's needs.

Some people in Sharon's situation stop socializing with friends, reduce their time at work, and often have increased conflict in their marital relationship as a result being less available to their spouse or partner. Although Sharon's situation represents an extreme scenario, guilt about having fun when not with the sick family member or not paying attention to the sick family member can be unrelenting. One spouse of a chronically ill patient told me that when she sees her friends and has moments when she is not worried about her husband, she becomes consumed with guilt and feels that she has done something wrong. Worry is often a way that people maintain a sense of ongoing care for the patient. Through worrying family members can maintain a sense that they are providing care for their loved one. This helps to maintain a sense of being connected to the patient, but can also help to manage guilt as well as increase sense of control. Although this control is often an illusion, not worrying makes the family members of patients feel as if they are being neglectful in some way; this can lead to or exacerbate intense guilt and shame.

When in the hospital, family members often approach me to commu-

patient, but it may also be that these family,

they have the time to think about how they are. In some instances, these family members say that they feel "fine" as they "are not the one who is sick." But clearly, in some instances, these family members aren't fine. In the hospital, nurses often report that family members have extreme anxiety as manifested by smothering patients and not allowing patients to achieve maximum independence or that they appear very depressed. I have heard of many instances in which family members of a patient suffer panic attacks during procedures that the patient is experiencing or of family members who ask nurses where they can get antidepressants for themselves while a patient is hospitalized. Certainly anxiety, sadness, and fear are normal responses when a loved one is ill, yet many family members seem to think that discussing their feelings is selfish or takes away from the care of the patient. Sometimes family members (particularly spouses and partners) feel guilty that their loved one was designated with a serious illness and not them. In other cases the feelings of helplessness and loss can get confused by external distractions, as in cases in which family members have irrational distrust in staff who are caring for a patient. Sharon's mistrust in the facility staff caring for her mother is one such example:

Sharon frequently complained that the staff did not pay enough attention to her mother. She eventually hired a caretaker to be with her mother several hours a day, even though her mother had frequent attendant care provided by the facility. Soon however, Sharon felt that the attendant she had hired was not attentive enough, and she fired this person and hired someone else. Eventually she was unhappy with the new attendant. The agency that she used refused to deal with her anymore because they felt she did not have any basis for her complaints about the attendants she fired. It seemed that every person who had contact with her mother was inadequate to take care of her. This was also an issue with her siblings whom she felt did not have her mother's best interests in mind. All of the intense worry about her mother began to take its toll on Sharon. She became depressed and gained 25 pounds. Her partner began to complain that she was never available and began to take vacations without her because Sharon felt that she could not leave her mother alone.

While it is common for family members to have concerns about the care of their loved ones, Sharon's preoccupation with her mother's care was destructive. She alienated herself from staff, physicians, and her partner. Her irrational mistrust was likely more about her complicated feelings for her mother than it was about ongoing care in the facility. It seemed that Sharon's loss of her mother from Alzheimer's dementia also caused her to think about how unavailable her mother was when she was young. Instead of thinking about the limitations of her mother's parenting, however, she became consumed with providing her mother with the best care possible and focused on others' inadequate performance in caring for her mother. Because this desire was rooted in her own losses, nothing ever felt good enough.

A serious illness in a family member understandably brings up a number of feelings. Children who are caring for ill parents are confronted with the fact that inevitably, their parent will die. For children who did not have good relationships with their parents, it can generate a wish for a last chance to get unfulfilled needs met. But when the child is in the position of caretaker, it is difficult to get these needs met. And while some children can eventually feel that they can make peace with their parent who was not able to fulfill all of their needs, others like Sharon focus their energy on health care professionals whom they perceive are not meeting the needs of their parent. One way of thinking about this is that family members who are overwhelmed by guilt, stress, and anxiety become externally focused as a way to avoid what they themselves are feeling. This kind of externalization by family members makes it difficult to take care of patients; physicians may feel tempted to avoid family members as well as the patients themselves. In talking with family members, physicians sometimes respond with anger, irritability, cool detachment, or even overt hostility. And while such responses are understandable, they usually inflame the family member more.

PROBLEMATIC SOCIAL SUPPORT

Family members often feel helpless when someone they love is ill.

patient, and although this may be partially true, sometimes being overly positive can be unhelpful to the patient. Patients often describe that they feel pressured to be positive; this often results in the sense that they cannot feel sad. One woman who had a mastectomy for breast cancer told me:

> "I feel so sad about how my body has changed and about what I have been through. But I can't really talk to my friends about it because they just tell me that I'm lucky. I know this is true, but I lost a part of my body. Shouldn't I be able to feel both lucky and sad?"

This woman's comments echo a frequent complaint I hear from patients about the support they receive from friends and family. They hear that they should feel lucky that they survived a serious illness, and this message suggests to patients that they do not have a right to feel sad. When patients are conflicted about how they feel in terms of their illness, when they feel both traumatized yet lucky, it can be very confusing to hear others' comments about being positive because it ignores the other aspect of the patients' feelings: the sadness and loss associated with illness.

Little empirical research has been done in this area, although the studies that do exist yield some interesting findings. One qualitative study sought to describe the nature of social support that is well intended, but is experienced as problematic for patients.[5] This study interviewed men and women who had been hospitalized for acute coronary events and asked them to describe interactions with family members which were perceived as problematic. Fifty-nine participants said that family members who engaged in excessive telephone contact, worrying and high expression of emotions, unsolicited advice, taking over, and the provision of advice without providing practical means for implementation were either excessive in meeting of their needs, incongruous with their needs, or contributing to negative feelings. Other studies have found that problematic support leads to reduced emotional well-being or depression. A study that looked at the disclosure patterns and social support of women with breast cancer found that women who disclosed their feelings about their illness less and who had unsupportive social interactions scored lower on measures of emotional well-being and were more likely to be depressed.[6] A study in the Netherlands surveyed two hundred and twenty-nine men and women with rheumatoid arthritis and found a correlation between problematic social support and depression.[7] Additionally, perceived problematic social support was correlated with increased reports of pain and more functional limitations. Fewer studies have looked at problematic social support and mortality in seriously ill patients. However, one study conducted in Germany found that problematic social support was associated with reduced survival in patients undergoing autologous bone marrow transplant.[8] However; this study did not find that positive social support had an association with increased survival. Additionally, survivors were more likely to receive interferon treatment and to receive psychotherapy. Nevertheless, these findings are consistent with other studies described in Chapter 1 suggesting the negative impact of poor social support.

It is difficult for physicians to know how to respond to family dynamics, especially because the nuances of these dynamics can be both subtle and complicated. Consider the following example:

> Jennifer is a 44-year-old female who had an extended hospital stay for complications following a routine surgery. Her husband, Aaron, was a physician in the hospital where she had her surgery. Staff noticed that interactions between the couple were tense and the couple were frequently heard to be arguing about his availability to her while she was in the hospital. Jennifer accused Aaron of being more concerned about taking care of his sick patients than with taking care of her, and Aaron often appeared distracted and irritable when talking with his wife. Although staff were concerned about the impact of these arguments on Jennifer, they said nothing because of Aaron's position.

This case raises a number of interesting issues. First, clearly the couple had ongoing issues related to Jennifer's resentment of Aaron's work

atient's cancer failed to go into remission and that there were no
ment options available for her. The couple told me that the physician
e in to the room early in the morning, woke the patient up and told
(before her husband had arrived) that her treatment had failed

iver this terrible news.

Most physicians need to develop emotional distance from the daily trau-
as that they see in order to continue to do their work. Dealing with fam-
y members often pulls the physician into highly emotional and sometimes
onflicted situations. These situations often require the physician to be
more available emotionally, which is not consistent with being emotionally
etached. These two roles, being detached in order to keep from getting
verwhelmed and being emotionally available for patients and families
strikes me as one of the more difficult challenges of being a physician.

In terms of practical suggestions, an obvious one is to attempt to spend
more time with families when they have questions. Part of the culture of
being a physician is that they have a lot of demands on their time and
spending extra time with families can feel stressful but will likely diffuse
tension and anxiety. As one physician described it: "When I am dealing with
families who are anxious and have a ton of questions, I just try to remind
myself that if I take care of this now, it will be easier in the long run. A extra
few minutes won't make a big difference in my day." Table 1 provides
additional suggestions for dealing with families of medically ill patients.

CONCLUSIONS

Illness requires patients and their family members to deal with feelings of
vulnerability. Feeling vulnerable is an issue for patients but in some ways
is more difficult for family members who are in the position of providing
care as there is an inherent expectation that care providers should not
express vulnerability. All relationships have problems; illness happens in
the context of these problems and often intensifies these problems, espe-

schedule. Second, it illustrates the complicated dynamics associated with
feelings of vulnerability that are inevitably associated with injury or illness. While Aaron may have been comfortable taking care of his sick
patients, taking care of his sick wife

the patient or family member is a VIP, hospital staff are often reluctant to intervene. In medical settings VIPs are often hospital staff, physicians, family of physicians, or people with prominent positions in the
community. Hospital staff and outpatient physicians often get anxious
when taking care of such patients and feel vulnerable that an error will
expose an inability to provide good care. Anyone trying to intervene with
Jennifer and Aaron could have been perceived by the couple as intrusive or
judgmental, and since Aaron was a physician in the hospital, staff likely did
not want to anger him. I have found, however, that in dealing with VIP
patients that a direct approach is often appreciated. Especially with health
care professionals who are on the receiving end of medical care, they are
often astute enough to know when staff are hesitant to communicate
concerns. Discussing concerns openly often diffuses tension and is a relief
to health care professionals (whether they are family members or patients)
as they then feel that they have permission to be treated like any other
recipient of health care, that they are real persons with real problems.

WHEN PATIENTS AND FAMILIES DON'T COMMUNICATE

Physicians often refer patients to a mental health professional when a patient
with a serious illness has not talked with family members about the illness. In
my experience such situations are surprisingly common and are concerning
to physicians who worry that a patient may not have adequate support or that
this may indicate that a patient may be in denial about the illness. These
instances can create difficult situations when patients are not talking to family members about the severity of their illness. I suspect that there may be
some cultural explanations for these kinds of situations, as some cultures

have strong prohibitions against talking about problems, including health problems. In addition to cultural variations in discussing problems, language barriers can present additional challenges. Consider the following example:

> Li is a 67-year-old man who emigrated to the United States from China when he was 28-years-old. He is newly diagnosed with stage 3B lung cancer, and his doctors have told his son that his prognosis is poor. Li doesn't speak English, so his physicians use his eldest son who attends appointments with him as a translator. In a follow-up visit in which he is to discuss treatment options, including radiation therapy, his son tells the physician that neither Li nor any other family members (which includes three other children) are aware of the severity of Li's illness and instructs the physician not to tell either Li's wife or any siblings about his prognosis. After the appointment however, the physician receives a call from Li's younger daughter who is eager to know the outcome of the last medical appointment.

Providing care in such situations for patients is difficult. Li's situation is complicated by the fact that he doesn't speak English and that the physician has to rely on a translator both to receive information from and to provide information to Li. The physician is in a bind. She or he may be unclear exactly what the patient's wishes are and unable to get more clear information from the patient. It is also unclear if the patient's son is in denial about the illness or he feels that he is protecting the patient and other family members by not disclosing the severity of Li's illness. If the physician is from a different culture than the patient, this kind of communication pattern may seem even harder to understand.

Another scenario occurs when patients are fully aware of their diagnosis and prognosis and do not tell family members about their illness. Some patients, perhaps partly as a denial of their illness or perhaps due to cultural reasons, feel that telling family members about their illness will be a burden. Some patients may provide a brief synopsis of their illness, but leave out important details regarding the impact of their illness. One patient, a man in his forties who had chronic graft vs. host disease following an allogenaic bone marrow transplant told me that his teenage son did not know about his ongoing physical symptoms of pain, gastrointestinal upset, and extreme fatigue. When I asked him why he hadn't discussed

this, he said that he didn't want to appear "weak' this man felt so embarrassed about how his illness able that the thought of discussing this with anyon

Physicians often feel that they have relatively littl in which patients and family members don't comm force family members to talk to one another, and questions about informed consent and medical de often difficult to know how aggressive to be in inter Sometimes reminding the patient and family that oper an important part of good care helps to reinforce the cian has the patient's best interest in mind. As discus some patients become very mistrustful when they are ill; physician feel helpless in knowing how to intervene.

SUGGESTIONS FOR FAMILY INTERVENT

Dealing with family members can be difficult and Physicians can feel an enormous amount of pressure to p tive answers to patients' family members, often when defin are difficult to provide. Some physicians avoid interactions discussions with family due to the ambiguous nature of ma illnesses. Research suggests that particularly when dealing v sions of end-of-life care, physicians are less likely to talk wi and family about their wishes for care.[9,10] Additionally, dealin intense emotions of family members can be complicated. As a c in different health care settings, I have been struck by the diffe staff and physicians' orientations to talk with patients and famili prognosis, palliative care, and the wishes of both patients and about care options. I suspect that the culture of different insti plays a role in this variability; some institutions tend to provide aggressive treatments for advanced diseases than others. Anothe able, however, is likely the personality of the physician. Physician themselves have difficulty with coming to terms with their own vu ability will likely have more difficulty talking with patients and fam especially when they need to deliver bad news. One situation that ex plifies this was a situation in which I was called in to talk with a husba and wife (the wife was the hospital inpatient) after they were told th

Table 1. Strategies for dealing with family members

Difficulty	Strategy
Conflict among family members	Acknowledge that underlying conflict tends to get worse durin~ ' illness
	...y person who ...sible for communicating to others
...y at the physician	Try to arrange meeting with family, or communicate availability (Anger is often diffused when physicians do not appear as if they are avoiding the family)
Family member is micromanaging	Provide information regarding patient's condition (in writing if possible) and resources where they can find out more information (This helps to increase sense of control)
Family provides problematic support	Encourage patient and family to talk about what kind of support patient finds useful

cially when illness becomes chronic. Dealing with the emotions of family members can be difficult for physicians, who may not be comfortable with the intense emotions that can get expressed by family members. After all, physicians are in the constant role of care provision, which is a role in which expressing vulnerability is not encouraged. Although not all family members express strong emotions, when they do or when the illness requires emotional conversations (e.g., talking about palliative care or advance directives), physicians are pulled into a role that may differ from what they are used to. This conflict is one of the many that makes practicing medicine difficult. Yet intervening proactively with patients' family members not only wards off potential problems, it can also make the work of physicians more rewarding.

REFERENCES

1. National Family Caregivers Association. *Caregiver Survey* 2000. Kensington, MD: National Family Caregivers Association; 2000.

2. Vanderwerker LC, Laff RE, Kadan-Lottick NS, McColl S, Prigerson HG. Psychiatric disorders and mental health service use among caregivers of advanced cancer patients. *J Clin Oncol.* 2005;23:6899–6907 [Epub 2005 Aug 29].

3. Pinquart M, Sörensen S. Differences between caregivers and noncaregivers in psychological health and physical health: a meta-analysis. *Psychol Aging.* 2003;18:250–267.

4. Pinquart M, Sörensen S. Ethnic differences in stressors, resources, and psychological outcomes of family caregiving: a meta-analysis. *Gerontologist.* 2005;45:90–106.

5. Boutin-Foster C. In spite of good intentions: patients' perspectives on problematic social support interactions. *Health Qual Life Outcomes.* 2005;3:52.

6. Figueiredo MI, Fries E, Ingram KM. The role of disclosure patterns and unsupportive social interactions in the well-being of cancer patients. *Psychooncology.* 2004;13:96–105.

7. Riemsma RP, Taal E, Wiegman O, Rasker JJ, Bruyn GAW, van Paassen HC. Problematic social support in relation to depression in people with rheumatoid arthritis. *J Health Psychol.* 2000;5:221–230.

8. Frick E, Motzke C, Fischer N, Busch R, Bumeder I. Is perceived social support a predictor of survival for patients undergoing autologous peripheral blood stem cell transplantation? *Psychooncology.* 2005;14:759–770.

9. Boyle DK, Miller PA, Forbes-Thompson SA. Communication and end-of-life care in the intensive care unit: patient, family and clinicians outcomes. *Crit Care Nurs Q.* 2005;28:302–316.

10. Kahana B, Dan K, Kahana E, Kercher K. The personal and social context of planning for end-of-life care. *J Am Geriatr Soc.* 2004;52:1163–1167.

7

TRUST IN

"Medicine is not merely a science but an art. The character of the physician may act more powerfully upon the patient than the drugs employed."

—Paracelsus

Throughout history, populations have looked for people to take away their mental, physical, and spiritual troubles. Shamans, priests, folk healers, and psychic healers provided hope for people with problems. In the 5th century B.C., Western medicine offered additional help, although the majority of cures and symptomatic relief that physicians could provide were not really developed until the late 19th century with medical advances rapidly developing throughout the 20th century. Before accurate diagnosis and medicines, physicians relied largely on the force of personality to heal. Bedside manner was an essential component of the house call. With today's technological and scientific advances, physicians can offer patients cures to many of the most serious health problems. In cases in which patients cannot be cured, life can often be extended, sometimes without major impact to quality of life. In spite of all of these advances, however, the relationship between doctor and patient remains central to the work of doctoring. Although the fact that physicians today can offer an array of effective treatments could suggest that the relationship between doctor and patient is less important, an equally compelling argument can be made that the doctor–patient relationship is more important than ever. As described in Chapter 2, Western medicine has become depersonalized, and both doctors and patients feel increasingly devalued as a result of technological advances, managed care, and the sheer increase in the number of patients who live long enough to require medical care. These changes imply that the relationship between doctors and patients can offer a possibility to make medicine more personal and to increase not only patient satisfaction but also job satisfaction among physicians who take care of patients. There is also the possibility that the crucial nature of the doctor–patient relationship could be healing and that physicians who use their authority in a particular way may have an impact on patients beyond the medical treatments they offer. The importance of social support, described in Chapter 1, provides evidence for this hypothesis, as physicians are a crucial social contact and potential avenue for support for patients.

This chapter will deal with the nature of relationships in medicine. Trust between patients and physicians will be discussed in the context of ethnic and socioeconomic variables, and research will be reviewed that suggests that trusting relationships are associated with better outcomes. I will also discuss that the difficulties physicians face in feeling that they can impact patients and how this is another potential moderator of trust between patients and physicians.

TRUST AND COMMUNICATION

As described in Chapter 2, the culture of American medicine has changed drastically. Physicians are simultaneously valued and devalued. Managed care, technology, and patient expectations for a good quality of life all contribute to increased demands on physicians. Physicians of the current generation may be less satisfied with their careers than previous generations. Although the public can devalue physicians for a number of reasons (based on what we know about human psychology, it is expected that people will tend to devalue those in positions of authority) physicians are still elevated as unique and talented healers. Though there are many examples of the public's lack of trust in Western medicine, physicians are still granted a kind of supreme, if not magical, authority. Not only do most people recognize how long physicians need to be in school and receive training before they practice, but the wish to be magically healed is something that many people crave. Patients who are vulnerable in both medical and psychological treatments are subject to this wish. Patient

that although they know it

...p. A patient who was
...son exemplifies this:

> "I know he's the expert, and I need him to make my problem better. But still, I wish he was nicer to me and spent more than a minute or two discussing my problem. He will be cutting me open, after all."

For the patient to know that he or she needs the physician is a necessary, although not sufficient, criterion for a good relationship. Good relationships require reliance on a physician's expertise but also a sense of trust, a belief that the physician cares about the patient's well-being, and that the patient is seen not as an object, but as an individual with unique needs. A belief in a physician's competence is, of course, related to trust. But many patients also want their doctors to be caring, kind, and patient. Patients often describe that trust as associated with physicians spending time with them, listening to them, and answering their questions. This latter aspect is complicated. Honesty is expected by some patients but discouraged by others. Two brief examples illustrate this:

A man in his mid-fifties who was a blue-collar laborer described an interaction he had with his attending physician while in the hospital for a serious life-threatening illness. The patient had been quite aggressive with a female attending, and his behavior with female nurses was equally disruptive and disrespectful. The patient told me that his primary attending physician, who was a white man and slightly older than the patient, told him regarding his interactions with the female staff, "You don't have to be a jerk to everybody just because you are dying." While this comment sounds shocking and potentially upsetting, the patient (who obviously did not die) told me that his physician's honesty regarding his inappropriate behavior helped to "turn him around." The patient continued to have a good relationship with this doctor and thought very fondly of him.

A young woman with a strong religious background was diagnosed with metastatic cancer. Her prognosis was poor, and one of her physicians indicated this to her, although there was some hope in prolonging her life with chemotherapy. She told me that she did not want to see this doctor anymore and requested another physician who tended to be more positive with patients, even in cases in which there was little hope for survival. She said to me, "I don't want to hear anything bad. If someone gives me bad news, I don't want to speak to them. I need to be positive."

As these two vignettes show, the issue of trust in patient–physician relationships is extremely complicated and dependent on the individual personality of both patient and physician. This argues for the need for physicians to alter their style when dealing with different patients. Many physicians do this intuitively. Perhaps the physician in the first vignette had a sense that he could get away with such a comment with this patient. (Although another possibility is that the physician may have been simply speaking in anger because the patient had been disrespectful to his colleagues.) Regardless of the explanation, it is clear that different patients need different things from their physicians.

One aspect of trust is communication. As is evident from the above examples, patients have different needs regarding communication styles. Different patients have different preferences regarding how much health information they would like to receive and how much information they are able to retain. These factors, as well as physician communication styles, are related to the unfortunate fact that patients sometimes have very different ideas about their treatment, disease severity, and prognosis than their physicians.

In cancer patients, for example, a number of studies have found that patients report not being told of their prognosis and overestimate the likelihood of cure.[1] Other research reflects the lack of information that patients have or retain regarding medical procedures. A study conducted in the U.K. interviewed 350 patients who had undergone laparoscopy for abdominal pain and found that almost 27 percent of patients were either incorrect or did not know the surgical procedure that was performed.[2] Obviously, it is unclear from these studies whether physicians are not communicating effectively with patients or whether patients are not retaining information. However, it is a common complaint among patients that their physicians don't communicate effectively. Although this may be true in some cases, some patients do not (

...sion maker, family tensions, cultural differences, patient capacity in participating in such discussions, as well as the need to time such discussions appropriately.[4] My experience has reflected these findings. Family members may need more time to accept a poor prognosis especially if the patient's condition has deteriorated quickly. Tense and complicated family dynamics certainly complicate communication and decision-making.

Some patients cope with illness by wanting as much information as possible; others cope by following their doctors' orders and not asking questions. As the young woman in the above example illustrates, some patients make a conscious choice that they do want hear "bad news." While this latter style of coping may have short-term benefits, it can be problematic when patients are dealing with both acute and long-term side effects of treatments and the resulting changes in quality of life. In situations in which patients and physicians are making decisions regarding treatment, physicians may present the option that they determine is best for the patient and there may not be extensive discussions regarding side effects or possible adverse consequences of treatment. Additionally, patients may not be interested in this information at the time because they are interested in symptom relief. For example, a patient experiencing an acute asthma exacerbation may not be interested in the possible side effects of steroid therapy; she or he may simply be interested in symptom reduction. It is usually after treatment has been initiated and the patient's primary symptoms are gone that side effects are noticed. It is at this point that patients often remark that they did not realize the side effects of the medication or treatment. Rarely does this turn into a conflict with the physician however; most patients realize that they needed to choose treatment or continue to have symptoms. This can be a problem in some circumstances when patients perceive that they were not told about serious long-term consequences of treatment. Usually the more severe the intervention and consequences the more impacted the patient is and the more likely the patient is to mistrust their physician. For example, a number of patients who have undergone allogeneic bone marrow transplant and are living with chronic graft versus host disease often report to me that they were not prepared for the major impact their transplant has had on their physical functioning. Although in many of these cases patients were told about the potential effects of graft versus host disease (as I have been present for these discussions or talked with patients myself about this), the patient clearly feels ill prepared. One explanation may be that telling a patient about possible side effects and consequences of a treatment is very different than the patient actually experiencing these unwanted effects. Most of us can probably relate to the experience of knowing of an unwanted situation intellectually but still feeling ill prepared when it arrives. It is likely that patients need time to process all of the implications of an illness and that developing acceptance and insight regarding the severe life-changing effects of illness and treatment is a slow and gradual process. Unfortunately, slow and gradual awareness is often inconsistent with the realities and demands of modern medicine. This discrepancy between the time people need to accept and retain information and how quickly decisions sometimes need to be made is another area of conflict that makes practicing medicine difficult and that threatens trust between patients and medical professionals.

Patient–physician communication is a complicated process that involves the physician's willingness to expend time and energy in imparting medical information as well as the patient's willingness and ability to receive information. A study that illustrates the importance of both patient and physician input in medical consultations found that patients who engaged their physicians through asking questions, expressing concerns and negative feelings, and being assertive were more likely to receive facilitative communication from physicians.[5] This study found that women, Caucasians, and those with more education were more likely be active in their care, which may reflect cultural differences, physician comfort with certain patient populations, as well as patient expectations of an active and communicative relationship with their physician. The study indicates that some patients (white, educated women) may feel entitled to more direct and active contact with their physicians and may also reflect the fact that some patients do not expect or feel entitled to that kind of contact with their physician. Other research indicates that a physician's style of com-

a movement away from the paternalistic practice of medicine in which physicians are blindly deferred to is probably better overall for physicians and patients, some patients prefer to be less active in their care. Ethnic, cultural, and socioeconomic issues as well as cohort differences may play a role in this and will be discussed in the next section. Additionally, it is also important to reiterate the impact of patient tolerance for information. Thinking about medical problems is difficult for many patients, and the psychology of illness is complicated. The reality of bodily failure is overwhelmingly painful for some patients, and discussing problems with their doctors can bring up realities patients may not be ready to face, especially patients who are seriously or terminally ill. In such situations, a physician may need to be patient and monitor patient behaviors and willingness to talk about treatment and prognosis. Relationships, including those between patients and physicians, need time to develop.

TRUST AND ETHNICITY

It has been speculated that there may be differences between ethnic and socioeconomic groups in terms of levels of trust of physicians. The Tuskegee experiments that began in the U.S. in the 1930s and continued for four decades, in which African American men were deliberately misinformed and denied access to treatment for syphilis by the U.S. Public Health Service as a way to study long-term effects of the disease, are often thought to be partly responsible for potential mistrust in the medical system among blacks. While the Tuskegee experiments would seem like reasonable justification for African Americans and possibly other ethnic groups to mistrust the American medical establishment, not all research has found that African Americans trust their doctors less than Caucasians do.[7–9] Other research, however, has found that African Americans and other ethnic minorities tend to trust their physicians less and are less satisfied with medical care.[10–12]

A moderating variable to explain these discrepant research findings may be class. Although there is little research on the impact of class among all ethnic groups and trust in medical settings, one hypothesis is that persons who are minorities and from low economic backgrounds are more susceptible to lower trust in medical encounters. Like most professional disciplines in the U.S., medicine has historically been a career chosen by white persons from upper class backgrounds. Even though this has changed in recent years with more physicians representing diverse ethnic and class backgrounds, the medical encounter is one in which often persons from low economic status come into contact with staff and physicians who are economically better off. This interaction of persons from lower class backgrounds with those from higher-class backgrounds is one we often take for granted, but patients are often aware of these differences. This may explain in part why some patients perceive that their physicians are subjecting them to medical tests and procedures solely for financial gain. A sense of being used as a way to make money is one aspect of feeling objectified, which persons who are economically disadvantaged may be more subject to. One patient who grew up poor and now lives a modest, lower-middle-class background described feeling suspicious when his physician told him he needed surgery for his hernia. He said:

> "I don't want any more surgery. My doctor told me that the surgeon called him to tell him that he thinks I should do this, but how am I supposed to know if the doctors aren't just using me so that they can make more money off of me? I feel fine, so I don't get why they have to do this to me."

Though it may be tempting to define such comments as overly suspicious or even paranoid, the differences in class between doctors and physicians are a problem for some patients. Persons from a higher socioeconomic class have resources to check out physician advice. They also are likely feel more entitled to ask questions, clarify information, and inquire about other treatment options. Persons without these resources are more dependent on physicians for their knowledge and expertise; this dependence can be overwhelmingly frightening and make trust in the physician–patient relationship more elusive.

... _p ...., patients who trusted their physicians and felt that their physician knew them well were more adherent. Another study looked at the likelihood of purchasing medications for populations likely to be nonadherent with medications due to economic pressures.[13] This study of over 900 Veterans Affairs patients with diabetes found that patients who had low trust in their physicians were more likely to forgo medications when cost was high. Although patients with depression were also found to be less likely to be adherent with medications, this study suggests a moderating impact in the physician–patient relationship. Other studies have found that patients with HIV infection as well as low back pain have better outcomes and increased adherence when patients trust physicians more and when the patient and physician have collaboratively discussed the treatment plan.[14,15]

In attempting to gain a better understanding of the nature of trust, it has been found that when a physician spends more time with a patient, the patient reports a higher level of trust.[9,16,17] Other behaviors that are associated with increased trust are active listening on the part of the physician, the provision of emotional support, providing information without the use of medical jargon, and asking for the patient's input in medical decisions.[12,15,17,18]

Since patient agreement of a treatment plan is associated with increased trust and likely with adherence, this raises the question of how to obtain patient agreement. Physicians are constantly making suggestions to patients about behavioral changes that need to be made, and some patients do not follow this advice. One could imagine that telling patients all day to change certain behaviors only to see that relatively few of these patients will actually follow this advice would lead to a sense of hopelessness and futility.

I was recently at a talk for primary care physicians on chronic obstructive pulmonary disease (COPD) given by a pulmonologist, and the internists in the group expressed frustration at hearing outcome data for these patients. They questioned, in effect, that since these patients won't stop smoking, what is the point in sitting through an hour lecture on COPD? The outcome of COPD is poor, as these physicians were well aware. I can appreciate this frustration. Part of what physicians do is to treat the results of behaviors that patients know are not good for them and yet persist in. These unhealthful behaviors include drinking alcohol excessively, using illegal substances, smoking cigarettes, overeating, and not exercising. Patients who won't stop these behaviors could potentially erode the level of trust that physicians have in their patients. It also could affect the level of impact that the physician feels that they have.

As the reader likely knows, there are health care models in place that integrate social workers, lay health care workers, nurses, and mental health workers into the care of patients, especially those in disadvantaged communities. In the U.K., there are many counselors on site in general practitioner offices. Although these programs are beneficial and increase patient satisfaction, the long-term effects of such programs are unclear.[19] However, having a multidisciplinary team reduces the stress associated with treating such patients, allows physicians to get help with treating mental health and social problems, and provides other avenues for long-term relationships that can be helpful for such patients.

It is difficult for physicians to provide advice that is ignored. Physicians seem to handle this issue in different ways. Many physicians use patient-centered approaches and hope that over time patients change their behaviors. Some physicians become frustrated, which leads to detachment, professional dissatisfaction, and burnout. Part of the frustration among physicians seems to be related to the responsibility associated with being a physician. Responsibility is a double-edged sword. On the one hand, physicians are in a unique position to powerfully impact patients lives. Conversely, physicians are not ultimately responsible for patient behaviors and choices. These two seemingly discrepant realities can be in conflict with one another. Medical students often exemplify this conflict. When they first begin to see patients, they express a lot of confusion regarding their responsibility, at times feeling overly responsible for their patients' behaviors and outcomes. At other times they feel helpless and resentful regarding their inability to impact patients' outcomes. This bind is common, and experience helps to reduce some of this confusion, but even for experienced physicians this dilemma is difficult. For example, in a recent conversation with a physician about a patient that h̲͟.̲.̲ serious health p̲r̲o̲b̲l̲e̲m̲

[text obscured]

̲.̲.̲.̲ ̲r̲e̲g̲a̲r̲d̲i̲n̲g̲ the ways he has ̲.̲.̲ ̲t̲h̲e̲r̲, she said she is very aware that her refusal to change has been her responsibility. Ironically, the fact that she sought out therapy (on her own, without her physician telling her to see someone) was an indicator that she had been listening to him. She came to see me because of her concerns that she hadn't been taking care of herself and while in therapy started a weight loss program and reduced her drinking significantly. This story illustrates that while physicians may feel that they have little impact on patients the true impact of the unique patient–physician relationship is often underappreciated.

CONCLUSIONS

Trust is important for both patients and physicians. Patients who trust their physicians are more satisfied and compliant. Physicians are in a unique position to provide social support to patients, and the long-term nature of many patient physician relationships allows time for trust to develop in ways that can help patients physically and emotionally. While most of the research addresses the importance of patient trust, there is little discussion in the literature of physician trust in their patients. Patients who are nonadherent and those who simply cannot change problematic health behaviors threaten to erode trust on the part of physicians. Therefore, it seems that part of the work of being a physician involves some acceptance and understanding about the inherent difficulties involved with impacting patient change. It seems to me that a balance is required between physician sense of responsibility and the detachment needed to avoid feeling overwhelmed. In other words, there are limits to what physicians can provide. Although physicians cannot make patients magically change their unhealthy behaviors, the relationship between doctors and patients remains extremely important and can have a powerful impact for many patients. However, the importance of this relationship places another level of pressure on physicians especially when the relationship between the doctor and the patient is poor, when the patient is nonadherent, or simply when the physician does not like or cannot understand the patient. Some of these situations will be addressed in the next chapter.

REFERENCES

1. Hagerty RG, Butow PN, Ellis PM, et al. Communicating prognosis in cancer care: a systematic review of the literature. Ann Oncol 2005;16:1005–53.
2. Murphy SM, Donnelly M, Fitzgerald T, et al. Patients' recall of clinical information following laparoscopy for acute abdominal pain. Br J Surg 2004; 91:485–88.
3. Hack TF, Degner LF, Parker PA. The communication goals and needs of cancer patients: a review. Psycho-oncology 2005;14; 831–45.
4. Anslem AH, Palda V, Guest CA, et al. Barriers to communication regarding end-of-life care: perspectives of care providers. J Crit Care 2005; 20:214–23.
5. Street RL, Gordon HS, Ward MM, et al. Patient participation in medical consultations: why some patients are more involved that others. Med Care 2005;43:960–69.
6. Makoul G. Perpetuating passivity: reliance and reciprocal determinism in physician patient interaction. J Health Communication 1998;3:233–59.
7. Trachtenberg F, Dugan E, Hall MA. How patients' trust relates to their involvement in medical care. J Fam Prac 2005; 54(4):344–52.
8. Mousley-Williams A, Lumley MA, Gillis M, et al. Barriers to treatment adherence among African American and white women with systemic lupus erythematosus. Arthritis and Rheumatism 2002; 47(6):630–38.
9. Friscella K, Meldrum S, Franks, P et al. Patient trust: is it related to patient centered behavior of primary care physicians? Med Care 2004: 42(11):1049–55.
10. Doescher MP, Saver B.G. Franks P, et al. Racial and ethnic disparities in perceptions of physician style and trust. Arch Fam Med 2000; 9:1156–63.
11. Safran DG, Taira DA, Rogers WH, et al. Linking primary care performance to outcomes of care. J Fam Prac 1998: 47(3):213–20.
12. Keating NL, Gandhi TK, Orav J, et al. Patient characteristics and experiences associated with trust in specialist physicians. Arch Intern Med 2004; 164:1015–20.

13. Piette JD, Heisler M, Krein S, et al. The role of patient-physician trust in moderating medication adherence due to cost pressures. Arch Intern Med 2005; 165:1749–55.

14. Schneider J, Kaplan SH, Greenfield S, et al. Better physician-patient relation

care experiences related to trust satisfaction and considering changing physicians? J Gen Intern Med 2002; 17:29–39.

18. Tucker CM, Herman KC, Pedersen TR, et al. Cultural sensitivity in physician-patient relationships. Med Care 2003; 41(7):859–70.

19. Bower P, Rowland N, Mellor Clark J, et al. Effectiveness and cost effectiveness of counseling in primary care. The Cochrane Database of Systematic Reviews 2002; Issue 1 Art No.: CD001025. DOI: 10.1002/14651858.CD001025.

8

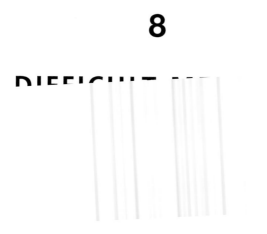

"*In this world there are only two tragedies. One is not getting what one wants, and the other is getting it.*"

—Oscar Wilde

Thus far I have been discussing a number of challenges that physicians face with patients, this chapter is more directly about what some physicians might refer to as "problem" or "difficult" patients. The term *difficult patient* sounds pejorative. Nonetheless, such patients exist and are experienced by physicians as a problem to manage. In the hospital, a difficult patient may receive a diagnosis of borderline personality disorder; many readers are familiar with such patients who "split" the treatment team. (This generally refers to the behavior of seeing one or more practitioners as benevolent and kind and others as bad, and attempting to align with those perceived as good and vilify those perceived as bad.) Although patients with borderline personality disorder are difficult to manage and represent a kind of caricature of difficult patients, physicians face other, more common difficulties while attempting to care for their patients. Difficult patients tend to use a lot of physician resources, both in terms of actual time spent with them, as well as expenditure of emotional energy. These patients include those who are noncompliant, angry, or disruptive to the patient–physician relationship and those who appear to be abusing medications or have psychosomatic complaints. This chapter will describe some common problems encountered with such patients, identify some of the psychological dynamics within these patients, and discuss interventions.

NONCOMPLIANCE

Noncompliance, which is often now referred to (in an attempt to sound less paternal and pejorative) as nonadherence,* is a common and frustrating problem. Not following the directions of a physician involves not stopping or reducing problematic health behaviors, not taking medications as prescribed, and not responding to physician advice and suggestions. Patients articulate different reasons for not following physician advice; these reasons can range from forgetting what was discussed with the physician, not agreeing with recommendations, not believing in the efficacy of treatment, resistance in arranging follow-up visits, time constraints, and the wish to avoid adverse effects of medications. Physicians are in a bind with a patient who is noncompliant because they are pulled into the position of convincing the patient to take care of himself or herself. One physician described her role in providing ongoing care to patients as being a "salesman trying to promote health; they either buy it or they don't." While this analogy is compelling in some ways, being a physician is not entirely like a being a salesman. If a customer doesn't buy a coat, the salesman doesn't have to worry that the customer will present to the salesman with an illness because he or she did not buy the coat for cold weather. Nor does the salesman have to treat the ill customer. The fact is, when patients do not follow physician advice, they place themselves at risk for further health problems, and the physician will be expected to care for the patient who becomes ill. Consider the following case example:

> John was a 26-year-old male who received a solid organ transplant. He did well during his hospitalization, although he did voice difficulty about leaving after his long hospital stay as he had become accustomed to being cared for by the physicians and nurses. Although he had trouble leaving the hospital, once he was out, he failed to attend many of his

---

* I will use the terms *nonadherent* and *noncompliant* synonymously.

follow-up appointments with his physicians. When he did attend, he made it clear that he did not want to see his doctors. Additionally, he was inconsistent in taking his medications. He presented in the emer-

immune system. Ultimately this involved him needing more care and more extensive contact with his providers. Different staff tried different methods to get him to follow his medication regimen as well as other post-transplant recommendations. Pleading, threatening, and discussing the consequences of his poor self-care were ineffective.

Although it could be argued that one's treatment of their body is a private and personal matter, as the example of John illustrates, once patients are part of the health care system their treatment of their bodies becomes something that others are invested in. Physicians, nurses, and other staff who are involved in patient care have an investment in patients' health. This seems to be particularly true in cases in which a patient has received extensive treatment or has utilized rare resources such as solid organs.

The research suggests that nonadherance to medical advice is common. Some estimates indicate that almost half of all medical patients in the United States do not adhere to medical advice regarding the prevention of disease or the treatment of both acute and chronic conditions.[1,2] In specific populations, nonadherence is high. For example, studies suggest that up to 40 percent of HIV patients, 20 percent to 40 percent of renal transplant patients, 20 percent of heart transplant patients, and 19 percent to 26 percent of patients being treated for osteoporosis do not take their medications as prescribed.[3–6] Depression is a risk factor for noncompliance in medical patients. A recent metaanalysis found that depressed patients are three times more likely to be noncompliant with treatment recommendations.[7] Low socioeconomic status combined with being a member of a racial or ethnic minority has also been associated with less medication adherence.[8] Lack of social support and less satisfaction with social support has been linked with noncompliance in transplant as well as HIV patients.[9–11] Certainly one can imagine that not having support, perhaps especially in the context of being economically disadvantaged or marginalized due to race would make it more difficult to pay attention to health concerns. Again, the care of one's body, although private in many ways, becomes a shared matter in the context of relationships. Family, close friends, and partners are also invested in the health of those they care about. They can help to remind patients to take medications and to follow physician advice, but relationships also serve to reinforce that a patient's health is valuable, because the patient himself is valuable. When this is lacking, self-care may slip away. Let us return to John.

John was a first-generation child of immigrant parents who came from an Asian country. He lived with his parents, and they were poor. His mother worked in a factory that makes clothes (an older sister told me that she worked in a sweat shop), and John's father did construction work when he could find jobs. When I spoke with John about his not taking his medication I asked him if there was anyone at home that could help remind him. He laughed and said, "My parents are having trouble taking care of themselves and my younger sisters, how could you expect that they could have time to remind me to take my medicine?" John was also preoccupied with taking care of himself financially. He wanted to move out but couldn't afford it. He had tried attending college courses but found that he got sick due to his weak immune system. He wanted to go to college so he could get a professional job, but he also wanted to go to work so that he could be independent and afford to live on his own. Attempts at working also failed as his health prevented him from being able to work in any job consistently.

Clearly John's lack of support and his own preoccupation with his economic situation made it difficult for him to focus on his health. While John's difficulty attending to his health was understandable, it was frustrating for his physicians who were less concerned about John's vocational and economic functioning and (understandably) more concerned with keeping John alive long enough to be able to entertain these worries. This raises an important difference in vantage points between some patients and physicians. Physicians may be sensitive to all kinds of racial, economic, and psychosocial stress, yet they have the task of prioritizing the health of their patients. In patients who are seriously ill, this often means focusing on the interventions and treatments that will keep patients alive. Patients on the other hand, may have other priorities. Not only is it normal to take health for granted to some extent (as discussed in Chapter 3) health may also feel like less of a priority when there are other pressing concerns. An example concerning physicians may further illustrate this point.

...appointments and not taking medications.

Yet, one wonders how seriously ill patients are able to avoid doing the necessary activities that will prolong life and will improve quality of life. Depression is likely to be a mediating variable as depression not only causes the loss of energy (anergia) that might be employed toward self-care but also reduces one's sense of self-worth. Additionally, people who are depressed often feel guilty, and this guilt can manifest itself in medical patients as feeling as if they deserve their illness. I often hear depressed patients speculate about whether they have been subject to the punishment of illness because of an imagined crime. (In some cases patients have to work really hard to conjure up what they may have done wrong. For example, a man with prostate cancer recently told me that he had spent a lot of time thinking about how he got cancer. In the absence of any major wrongdoing that he could identify, he wondered if a conflict he had with a neighbor years ago could explain it!) When one feels that one is being punished deservedly it may make it even harder to take care of oneself and to prioritize health. Depression also involves suicidal ideation. This suicidality may be active and involve specific thoughts and plans about taking one's own life. In my experience, however, this type of suicidality is relatively rare in medical patients. What is more common, however, is what I think of as passive suicidality; not caring for oneself and then waiting for the consequences. Patients who are lonely and isolated seem particularly at risk for passive suicidality. This behavior is often difficult to talk with patients about as feeling suicidal may not be something that patient is actively aware of. Discussions about not taking care of oneself and related self-destructive behaviors can be experienced by patients as blaming and unsympathetic. For example:

John told me about an interaction he had with one of his physicians who confronted him about his not attending appointments and not taking his medications. John said that the physician told him that his behavior would kill him eventually and then implied that perhaps John wanted to die. John vehemently denied this claim and then repeated how happy he was to have received his transplant. While the physician was likely correct in his interpretation of John's behavior, John seemed to have felt "caught" by his doctor. This, in combination with his own denial of his depression and passive suicidal behavior, caused him to feel the need to sound grateful when speaking with his doctor.

Patients often feel guilty for being noncompliant. Although this guilt may not result in patients becoming more compliant, it does often result in patients feeling the need to present as agreeable when meeting with physicians and is also related to patients' avoidance of their physicians.

As is evident from the above discussion, noncompliance takes place in the context of several relationships: the relationship with the physician and relationships with family, spouses, and friends. Noncompliance is important because it has the potential to invoke a number of intense and negative feelings in those who have a relationship with the patient. Feelings in the patient about the illness or about longstanding psychological issues can be experienced by others in relationship with the patient. Anger is one of these emotions. It is expected that physicians might get angry when patients don't follow advice or take medications, but this may also be indicative of anger that is experienced by the patient as well. (This type of dynamic can also be experienced with patients who are very sad: I once saw a young man in the hospital who had been a victim of a terrible, disfiguring accident. He appeared to be coping well, in fact he denied any feelings of sadness or loss. Yet, physicians and staff often left the patient's room crying, as if they absorbed his sadness from him!) Noncompliant patients may also have a lot of anger; creating a situation in which their physician is angry at them is one way (though nonproductive) that anger can get expressed. Consider John again:

John saw me intermittently for several years following his transplant. During one of our meetings he was describing a recent hospitalization. This hospitalization was not related to his transplant or due to immunosuppression. As he discussed this recent illness, it was clear that John felt despairingly toward his transplant doctors as he implied several times that they did not know what they were doing.

I was initially puzzled about this as they had little to do with his recent illness. It became clear that he felt very angry at his transplant doctors for all of his medical problems, his compromised quality of life, and because he was unhappy with his life in general. I then asked him if he thought that he didn't take his medication

quences, but the powerful attachments patients develop with those that care for them can create these kinds of emotional expressions. Sometimes identifying the anger can help improve adherence, as it eventually did in John's case. Psychotherapy was instrumental to this end as it turned out John had many other issues related to a disruptive family environment that contributed to his anger. Physicians are not often in the position to have such extended conversations with patients. When they are viewed as the instigators of the patients' physical problems, it is even harder for physicians to intervene. However, John's situation illustrates the powerful attachments patients develop with their doctors. At times the associations that patients develop because of this attachment can seem irrational. John's physicians saved his life, yet John felt they ruined it. John's anger was directed at the physicians probably in part because he had very few close attachments and he hadn't had a lot of experience with caring authority figures. Ironically, John's angry attachment to them and his noncompliance served the function of his having more contact with them. I came to appreciate that on some level John wanted more contact with his providers. When I knew John in the hospital, he told me when he was about to be discharged that he did not want to leave because he felt that the staff and the physicians were so caring. I eventually understood after learning more about his family situation that John had had very little contact with persons he felt cared about him. He grew dependent on this care, yet was angry that he needed these authority figures to meet his physical and emotional needs. By rebelling through not taking care of himself he ensured that he would continue to need his doctors.

Nonadherent patients are difficult for physicians to deal with, but the weight of a strong attachment can be used by physicians to positively impact patients. In my experience, physicians are often unaware how important they are to patients. The practice of medicine can feel devaluing in general, and a patient who misses appointments and does not follow physician advice can reinforce a physician's sense of being devalued. While it may be the case that some patients do not value their doctors, it seems to me that this is rarely the sole explanation for nonadherence. The self-destructive nature of noncompliance suggests the presence of a number of psychological issues, including depression. Addressing undiagnosed mood disturbances is one strategy to intervene with nonadherent patients. Also, telling the patient in a concerned tone rather than an angry one that his or her behavior is damaging sometimes helps patients to recognize the misguided nature of their behavior. Increasing patients' sense of control is also helpful. For example, one physician told me that she allows some patients to determine optimal doses of certain medications. She makes a point to tell patients that she trusts in their ability to know what is best. As discussed in the previous chapter, trust of physicians is associated with increased compliance. This intervention indicates that that physician trusts the patient and is likely to have a reciprocal effect, as well as the effect of strengthening the relationship. Other interventions that increase trust include active listening and empathy, as well as nondefensive acknowledgement of the patient's distress and sense of having been unfairly picked to become ill.

MEDICATION ABUSE AND ADDICTION

Physicians are in the unique position to prescribe controlled substances that have powerful physical and psychological effects. Benzodiazepines and opioids are among the medications that have the ability to manage anxiety and pain, respectively, but also have the potential for dependence, abuse, and addiction. Many patients use these medications responsibly. However, problems develop when patients require additional doses of these medications that exceed the physician's opinion of what is needed. Consider the following case example:

> Sara is a 28-year-old woman who works in an administrative position. She developed headaches that were deemed to possibly be of migraine classification and received opioids from her primary care physician to

manage her pain. Over the course of a couple of years, she increased her use of narcotics and had progressed to the use of a very strong opioid. Her physician referred her for psychotherapy when he became concerned that h...

...g... her to come in. ...he had trouble telling me why she came to see me, and in our initial interview never mentioned her headaches or her use of opioids. In fact, she denied any subjective psychological distress although alluded to living with her alcoholic father and feeling sorry for her mother who took care of him. Following our initial meeting, her physician told Sara that he would no longer prescribe her medications unless she received treatment for substance abuse. She came to see me again and was angry but also surprised by this recent declaration on the part of her physician. She said, "I don't get it. He gave me these medications for years, and now I am supposedly addicted. I took them because he told me to."

This case example illustrates an unfortunate situation concerning the use of opioids to treat chronic nonmalignant pain. She had become addicted to pain medication, and her physician who had prescribed these medications was concerned about the consequences. Patients who become addicted to pain medication or benzodiazepines often complain that they did not know that the medications could cause physiological dependence as well as psychological dependence. This latter term is now generally referred to as addiction to reflect the neurobiological correlates of addictive disease. Addiction is often defined as compulsive behavior to use a substance in the face of adverse consequences, not just the presence of withdrawal.[12] Abuse of medication is often defined as intentional use of medications (especially opioids) that is outside of a physician's prescription for a bona fide medical problem.[13]

The issue of patients' abuse and addiction to medications, particularly opioids, is complicated by increasing concern that pain is undertreated.

In recent years, pain physicians and pain societies have advocated for improved pain control including the development of guidelines for chronic pain management, which includes the use of opioids.[14] This shift to a more sensitive approach to managing pain makes it more difficult to address patients that do abuse pain medications. Clearly there are patients who have pain that is undertreated. I have observed this to be especially true in postsurgical patients who have been on narcotics presurgery and need higher doses of pain medications for postoperative pain. Physicians are understandably concerned, however, with prescribing high doses of opiates due to potentially adverse effects, including respiratory depression. Pain is a complex experience, however, and involves both neurological and emotional pathways, with anxiety often increasing a patient's experience of pain. The fact that some patients who are prescribed opiates for pain appear to use the medications to decrease anxiety could make physicians wonder if by prescribing narcotics for pain relief, if they are actually treating the pain or if they are treating another, perhaps insidious psychiatric condition. However, since pain also increases anxiety, it can be difficult to know what the patient's psychiatric condition really is.

Predicting addiction is difficult, and behavior that can appear to be drug-seeking may present in patients who are not addicted to opioids. For example, one study found that up to 20 percent of patients who did not meet criteria for addiction engaged in drug hoarding during periods of fewer symptoms, complaining about wanting more medications, requesting specific drugs, and being reluctant to change medication.[15] A prior history of substance abuse and anxiety is associated with abuse or addiction to pain medications.[16] In this study, these risk factors were thought to be mediated by beliefs that opiates are effective in treating chronic pain, that these medications improve mood, that higher functioning is associated with medication use, and a belief that higher amounts of narcotics are needed for pain control. Sara's situation reflected the above research findings:

Sara had symptoms of both anxiety and depression. She eventually told me that her family situation was quite difficult; yet she could not afford to live on her own. She also told me that she was suicidal and that she had thought of using her pain medication to end her life and that her disclosure of this to her primary care physician is what alarmed him and resulted in the referral to myself. Additionally,

Sara acknowledged that she did not feel that there were any other strategies for treating her physical and psychological pain. She felt trapped in her home situation and her low-paying job. She had few friends. In fact, her relationship with her physician was her primary source of social support. She was fond of him

Behavioral interventions are often recommended in dealing with such patients. Taking medications when one is addicted is powerfully reinforcing, both physiologically and psychologically. As we saw with Sara, she did not feel that she had a problem; at the time she saw me, she thought her only problem was that her doctor was threatening to take her medication away. Her physician, who prided himself on spending a lot of time with his patients, and who was constitutionally a kind, caring, and patient man, had spent countless hours tying to help Sara see that her use of her medications was problematic. Sara never agreed and continued to have minimal insight regarding her use of narcotics. Her physician eventually developed a contract with Sara outlining that in order to continue receiving her medication from him she needed to refrain from seeing other physicians (coordinating care with one prescriber is a common intervention with medication-abusing patients), agree to gradually lower her dosage, and switch to a less strong narcotic. The contract included that she get treatment for her anxiety and depression, whether through antidepressant treatment or psychotherapy. Sara initially agreed to the contract but was soon abusing opiates and requesting multiple prescriptions. Her physician referred her to a treatment program that specialized in treating patients with medical disorders who were addicted to medications. Sara refused this referral and switched physicians.

Although a (somewhat cynical) argument can be made that this outcome was positive for the physician who got rid of a difficult patient, the patient likely went on to another physician and repeated the same pattern, which makes this outcome less positive for the patient and the next physician. The helplessness evoked by difficult patients, especially those abusing substances, can cause physicians to feel that the only option is for the patient to leave. It is reasonable for patients who are on long-term opiates to be referred to pain clinics that specialize in treating such patients and that have multidisciplinary teams to help manage them. Patients who are addicted to medications, however, are in need of help from their physician to identify the problem, acknowledge that there are other psychosocial stresses associated with the medication use, and to help taper doses if appropriate. At times mental health professionals can aid in such interventions if the patient is willing.

ANGRY AND DISRUPTIVE PATIENTS

Although a number of patients develop anger after becoming ill, and anger can be construed as a normative response to illness, there are some patients whose anger is so primary that they alienate the professionals who are trying to take care of them. Consider the case of Raymond:

> Raymond was 53-years old and had developed symptoms consistent with liver disease. His abnormal liver function tests worried his physician who ordered a liver biopsy. When Raymond presented for his liver biopsy he refused any pain medication or an anxiolytic to help him through the procedure. The physician performing the procedure was puzzled and concerned; she did not want to do the procedure without offering some comfort for the patient. Yet, the patient insisted on doing the procedure without medications. The physician began the procedure and the patient stated that he would not go through the procedure and then, with considerable profanity, told the physician that he would not ever undergo this procedure, that he did not need it, and that she was unqualified to perform the procedure on him. The physician was stunned and angry and referred Raymond for a psychological evaluation before he was allowed any further treatment.

Raymond illustrates an extreme situation in which his disruptive behavior prevented him from receiving an important diagnostic test. When I met with him, it was evident that he actually had had a panic attack in response to his fear of being ill and his fear of being out of control during the procedure. Raymond met full criteria for panic disorder, and it was clear that his panic attack was associated with his aggressive behavior toward his physician. Although we often think of panic disorder as involving fear, a number of patients with panic reactions behave aggressively in response to their fear. One way of thinking about this is that anxiety and especially panic initiate the

when being taken care of. This can manifest itself as suspiciousness and paranoia:

Raymond ultimately received his liver biopsy. He did so without medication. When I asked him why he wouldn't take something for pain or anxiety, he said, "I am not taking any drugs. We don't really know what they do to us, what the long-term effects are. I am not going to be a guinea pig for those doctors to test out these drugs."

When paranoia presents in this way (in persons who were functional and not overtly paranoid before an illness), I often think it represents a kind of collapsing of defenses and coping mechanisms. In other words, the patient's normal ways of protecting himself and soothing his anxiety stops working. Paranoia is the result of these failed coping mechanisms as this internal psychological collapse makes it difficult to know who to trust in the external world.

It can be difficult to know how to intervene with angry and paranoid patients. Paranoid patients often spend a lot of time imagining what others are thinking, and they constantly have to monitor the environment in an attempt to watch for signs of danger. Since physicians are often the messengers of bad news as well as the purveyors of pain and discomfort through procedures, paranoid patients often view the physician as the enemy. What helps in these situations is if the physician can be as open as possible with the patient and by being open give the patient the sense that she has access to the physician's mind. For example saying to the patient, "Right now I am thinking . . ." or "I think we should proceed this way because . . ." Paranoid patients are soothed by feeling as if they have access to others' minds as this decreases the amount of information that they have to speculate about. In fact, in the hospital I often recommend that physicians and staff with more disinhibited and gregarious personalities take care of paranoid patients. Physicians and staff who are more reserved tend to make paranoid patients more suspicious, even if they are kind and well-intentioned people.

Another kind of angry patient is one who develops irrational ideas about the physician and becomes convinced that certain traits are attributable to the physician even when there is no evidence to support these assumptions. These assumptions make it difficult to for the physician to understand the patient. Consider the following example:

> Jessica is a 35-year-old woman who injured her spine while rock climbing. She needed surgery to repair damaged disks and consulted a reputable spine surgeon. The surgeon met with Jessica a couple of times to discuss the surgery, and a surgery date was set. Jessica cancelled the surgery date one day before the procedure saying that she had changed her mind. She then went to see the surgeon and said she wanted surgery after all. Her surgeon, puzzled and irritated, referred Jessica to me. Jessica told me that she liked her surgeon, who had spent a lot of time with Jessica. Yet, Jessica was convinced that her surgeon "didn't care enough about her." When I asked her what this meant, Jessica said that since she was allowing the surgeon to "cut her open" that it was crucial that she felt connected to him. Thus far the surgeon had spent more time on Jessica's case than he usually did with other patients, including a phone call with me in the evening to talk about her. Although Jessica may not have felt connected enough to the surgeon, it was clear the surgeon was connected to Jessica! It turned out that Jessica had very unavailable parents while growing up, and as she told me about her background, she described series of incidents in which she felt extremely vulnerable, but without any support from authority figures to help her feel safe. Although she had evidence that her surgeon did care about her, she needed almost constant reassurance from him that he did care.

Jessica's conflict about not feeling that others care for her and will help take care of her when she is vulnerable was played out with her surgeon. While some fear of a major surgery is normal, Jessica's fears were excessive; her need for constant reassurance from her surgeon was based on past experiences, not the present relationship with her doctor. This dynamic, in which patients develop ideas and feelings about a current relationship, but the feelings are more related to relationships that have taken place in the past is known as transf...

... available for her she had trouble believing that her surgeon really had her best interest in mind. Fortunately, her surgeon was sensitive to this dynamic and met with Jessica for an extended appointment to discuss the surgery and allay her fears. Jessica went on to have surgery and did well.

PSYCHOSOMATIC COMPLAINTS

Psychosomatic complaints, which I define as physical complaints that are in excess of organic findings, occur in patients who are physically healthy as well as in those who have chronic conditions. Surveys indicate that physicians have rated 7 percent to 25 percent of visits as unnecessary or trival.[18] Psychosomatic complaints are often associated with those who are well physically and are often attributed to mental health issues. However, in my experience, a small but significant number of patients who have chronic medical conditions or who have been treated and are in remission from serious medical conditions develop complaints that occur either in the absence of organic findings or are in excess of what might be expected in a given condition. Consider the following example:

> Joan is a 45-year-old woman who was born with a rare, but not life-threatening, autoimmune disorder. The disorder impacted the appearance of her skin through the presence of pigmented lesions. She was successfully treated with steroids for this disorder, but at different times throughout her life had to seek treatment due to flair-ups of her symptoms. The nature of her disease is unpredictable. She attempted to attribute her symptoms to a variety of causes including stress, but was unable

fully to ever isolate variables that might help her to identify contributing factors. When she came to see me, the symptoms of her autoimmune disorder were under control, but she had developed a fear that she had heart disease. She worried that she was having a heart attack and frequently presented to her physician with these concerns. Her physician did a full work-up and concluded that she did not have heart disease. In fact, she was quite healthy despite her autoimmune disorder. Joan was not satisfied with this assessment, however, and saw two other physicians for another opinion, who came to the same conclusion.

Joan was worried that she had heart disease although there was no evidence to support this fear. Patients with such worries frequently present to their primary care physician and take up a lot of physician time. Joan came to therapy at her physician's urging, but many patients with psychosomatic complaints refuse referrals for therapy because they feel that their issues are physical in nature. When such patients do present in a psychotherapist's office they are often resentful. Joan said:

> I am only here because my doctor told me to come. She's fed up with me and doesn't believe me; that's why she sent me. My problems are physical not mental. I don't need to see you.

Patients who have psychosomatic complaints often experience a referral to a mental health professional as a kind of insult, as well as a defeat. They feel with the utmost certainty that they have something physically wrong with them and that a referral to a mental health professional illustrates that the physician has given up on them. This perception is not necessarily unrealistic. In our country of very divided mental health and physical service provision, a referral to a mental health clinician can and often does indicate that the physician feels that there is nothing left to offer the patient except a mental health professional. Such patients value a physical explanation for their problems, and not receiving this is experienced as a failure either on the part of the physician to understand the problem or on the part of the patient to sufficiently convince the doctor of the reality of the problem.

How are we to understand the nature of psychological issues that arise in patients like Joan? From her physician's perspective, she is fine and does not need physical treatment. Obviously, in such cases it is reasonable to conclude that psychological factors are causing a psychosomatic response. When something is wrong, physically or mentally, patients often present to their physicians first. This is likely because patients have a relationship with their physician but also because of the idea that their problems must be physical

ᴵreating patients with psychosomatic symptoms is difficult and requires a lot of patience on the part of the physician. Helping to educate patients about the interaction between psychological issues and physical symptoms helps to normalize such symptoms and can make patients less defensive. Additionally, telling patients that their symptoms are real in spite of a lack of evidence of specific disease also helps patients feel less psychologically pathologized.

WHAT CAN DIFFICULT PATIENTS TEACH US? IMPLICATIONS FOR MEDICAL PRACTICE

Difficult patients are those that require additional time, energy, and resources, largely due to psychological problems. When patients are distressed, angry, or disruptive, it can be difficult for physicians to be sympathetic, especially when patients have what appear to be irrational ideas about the physician. Yet, for those of us in positions of authority, an acknowledgement of patient's feelings toward us, even if they are negative feelings, can be extremely useful. This is likely what makes psychotherapy useful for some patients. In the process of therapy, patients develop irrational ideas about the therapist. This dynamic involves transference, as described previously; patients develop ideas about therapists that may in fact be feelings based on other relationships from the past. Part of the training of many therapists involves being sensitive to transference dynamics and allowing the patient to express his or her thoughts without the therapist passing judgment. Physicians often do not receive this kind of training, as the culture of medicine in the United States does not support such approaches. There is an inherent expectation in our country that the body is separate from the mind; when mental and emotional dynamics present themselves in medical settings they are often viewed as unusual or aberrant. With such a system in place, it is difficult for even the most thoughtful and sensitive physicians to allocate time and energy to psychological issues. Difficult patients seem to demand this energy. They bring to our attention the lack of integration in our health system and force us to summon up additional resources to take care of them.

Although psychiatry is integrated into medical school curriculums, its principles remain outside of how many physicians practice. This may be in part due to the prevalence of biological psychiatry that is taught in many medical schools, an approach that does not emphasize a wide range of psychotherapeutic interventions. Other countries have attempted to integrate psychotherapeutic approaches, including psychoanalysis in medicine. Germany is the most noteworthy of these countries, and physicians there have been striving toward an integrative form of medicine, referred to as *psychosomatic medicine,* for decades.[19,20] In fact, physicians who practice in psychosomatic clinics receive training in psychotherapy.[21] Although in the United States there may be an appreciation of psychological issues, there is more emphasis given to psychological issues, including unconscious conflicts (such as transference) in some German internal medicine practices.[22] Though the realities of practicing medicine in this country may preclude such approaches, it is useful to remember that difficult patients serve to remind us of the difficulties associated with an unintegrated health care system.

REFERENCES

1. DiMatteo MR. Enhancing patient adherence to medical recommendations. *JAMA.* 1994;271:79–83.
2. DiMatteo MR, DiNicola DD. *Achieving Patient Compliance.* Elmsford, NY: Pergamon Press Inc; 1982.
3. Deschamps AE, Graeve VD, van Wijngaerden E, et al. Prevalence and correlates of nonadherence to antiretroviral therapy in a population of HIV patients using medication event monitoring system. *AIDS Patient Care STDS.* 2004;18:644–657.
4. Morrissey PE, Reinert S, Yango A, et al. Factors contributing to acute rejection in renal transplantation: the role of noncompliance. *Transplant Proc.* 2005;37: 2044–2047.
5. Dew MA, Kormos RL, Roth LH, et al. Early post-transplant medical compliance and mental health predict physical morbidity and mortality one to three years after heart transplantation. *J Heart Lung Transplant.* 1999;18:549–562.

6. Tosteson AN, Grove MR, Hammond CS, et al. Early discontinuation of treatment for osteoporosis. *Am J Med*. 2003;115:209–216.

7. DiMatteo MR, Lepper HS, Croghan TW. Depression is a risk factor for noncompliance with medical treatment. *Arch Intern Med*. 2000;160:2101–2107

8. Kaplan RC, Ph... ... ... recipients. ...nspl Int. 2005;18:1072–1078.

11. Viswanathan H, Anderson R, Thomas J. Evaluation of an antiretroviral medication attitude scale and relationships between medication attitudes and medication nonadherence. *AIDS Patient Care STDS*. 2005;19:306–316.

12. Schnoll SH, Weaver MF. Addiction and pain. *Am J Addict*. 2003;12(suppl 2): S27–S35.

13. Compton WM, Volkow ND. Major increases in opioid analgesic abuse in the United States: concerns and strategies. *Drug Alcohol Depend*. Jul 2005 [Epub ahead of print].

14. Green CR, Wheeler JRC, LaPorte F, et al. How well is chronic pain managed? Who does it well? *Pain Med*. 2002;3:56–65.

15. Compton P, Daarakjian J, Miotto K. Screening for addiction in patients in chronic pain and "problematic" substance use: evaluation of a pilot assessment tool. *J Pain Symptom Manage*. 1998;16:355–363.

16. Schieffer BM, Pham Q, Labus J, et al. Pain medication beliefs and medication misuse in chronic pain. *J Pain*. 2005;6:620–629.

17. Jage J. Opioid tolerence and dependence–do they matter? *Eur J Pain*. 2005;9:157–162.

18. Wagner PJ, Hendrich JE. Physician views on frequent medical use: patient beliefs and demographic and diagnostic correlates. *J Fam Pract*. 1993;36:417–422.

19. Roelecke, V. Psychotherapy between medicine, psychoanalysis, and politics: concepts practices, and institutions in Germany, c. 1945–1992. *Med Hist*. 2004;48:473–492.

20. Schuffel W, Egle U. Psychosomatic education in West Germany. *J Psychosom Res*. 1983;27:9–15.

21. Lamprecht F, Schueffel W, Maoz B. Psychosomatic medicine and primary care in Germany. *Isr J Psychiatry Relat Sci*. 1998;35:97–103.

22. Nigrovic A. Psychosomatic medicine in Germany. *Advances* 1994;10:66–71.

9

"With health, everything is a source of pleasure; without it, nothing else, whatever it may be, is enjoyable . . . Health is by far the most important element in human happiness."

—Arthur Schopenhauer

Physicians, especially primary care physicians, are in the position to diagnose and treat a variety of mental health problems. Many patients with mental health problems seek the advice of their physician first. For example, some mental health problems can manifest themselves physically, and physicians are often the first to diagnose psychosomatic illnesses. Additionally, the long-term relationships that physicians have with their patients allow them to detect untreated depression and anxiety. Physicians can prescribe medications for the treatment of many psychological problems. However, not all mental health problems are successfully treated in the primary care setting, and referrals to mental health providers are then necessary. This chapter will address issues associated with referring to a mental health professional. Referrals to mental health clinicians can be complicated for many reasons. First, many patients are quite sensitive to the meaning of a referral to a mental health professional. Another issue is that since mental health clinicians and physicians have different training, communication across disciplines can be difficult. These issues will be addressed first; then I will discuss how and when to refer patients for mental health treatment.

DIFFICULTIES IN REFERRALS FOR MENTAL HEALTH

Referrals within the specialty of medicine are routine and relatively uncomplicated. When physicians refer to other physicians, they are referring to other professionals with the same philosophical training. Additionally, these referrals often go unremarked by patients as they expect that seeing one physician may lead to a referral to a specialist physician. In contrast, referrals to mental health providers can be complicated because there is often a stigma associated with seeing a mental health provider. The stigma of mental health issues in medicine and in the United States culture as a whole makes referring to a mental health professional difficult for both health professionals and patients. Patients commonly worry that seeing a mental health professional indicates that they are "crazy." Thinking and talking about emotions is difficult for many people, and the intensity of feelings that arise when talking about their mental health can make them worry that they are crazy. Additionally, many people worry that merely talking about problems will make them become crazy. In addition to these concerns, there are other difficulties in making mental health referrals that are specific to medical practitioners.

Sometimes, being referred to a mental health professional suggests to patients that the physician feels nothing else can be offered medically. For example, patients often say to me that they are seeing me because their doctor "has nothing left to offer." Sometimes this is the case, for example, when a patient has a number of psychosomatic complaints and the physician has ruled out physical causes. When physicians refer patients for mental health services with the explicit or implicit message that they have nothing else left to offer, it can have the unintentional effect of devaluing both the patient and the mental health professional. Patients feel they are relegated to the mental health profession because the real doctor can't help them. Although this is often not the intended message, patients can experience it this way nonetheless, probably in part due to the stigma associated with mental health services. Additionally, when patients are referred to a mental health professional, it usually indicates that some deviation from the normative patient/physician interaction has occurred. For example, if a patient starts crying when talking to a physician in the hospital and/or seems as if she is not coping with her illness, this may result in a referral to a mental health professional. Though it is expected that a patient in distress could be referred to someone who has more time and

...when mental health services and physical health services are offered separately. As discussed in Chapter 2, the practices of mental health and medicine reflect different professional identities, training, and philosophies. Although psychiatric consult/liaison services in hospitals and the presence of mental health providers in primary clinics are notable exceptions to the usual separate practice of these disciplines, the majority of physicians do not have regular contact with mental health providers. A common complaint that I hear from physicians is that mental health providers do not speak the same language as they do. Indeed this is often the case. I remember the difficulties I had when I was in training and trying to understand psychological concepts myself and then trying to impart these concepts in a useful way to physicians. I would try to describe what I thought was going on with a patient without sensitivity to the way a physician might view it and would be met with a blank stare or simply be told that I didn't know what I was talking about! Now when I teach and train mental health professionals in medical settings, I emphasize the need to understand medical terminology, basic medical pathology, and medical treatments. Mental health clinicians need to become familiar with the culture of medicine in order to practice effectively within it. A mental health provider working in a medical setting needs to understand psychological theories, some aspects of medicine, and the basic philosophical assumptions that are part of medical science. Yet this understanding is often not sufficient for working effectively with physicians. Psychiatrists are physicians but often have the same difficulties communicating effectively with physicians as nonphysician mental health providers. The fact that the body and the mind are viewed separately and (with the exception of biological psychiatry) theories of mental health and physical functioning have different philosophical assumptions, likely explains some of these difficulties. It may also be that while mental health providers need education regarding some aspects of medicine, physicians may understand little about mental health issues and psychological theories. Although medical schools require rotations in psychiatry, this training is often in biomedical approaches to psychiatry, which don't address many of the mental health issues that physicians confront when they are in practice. What is often minimally addressed in these curricula is an understanding of personality functioning, character pathology, family dynamics, and therapeutic interventions other than cognitive behavioral approaches. Since psychiatry is a specialized field and requires a four-year residency, it makes sense that these issues cannot be fully addressed in medical schools. Nevertheless, the language of mental health providers and those of physical health providers are different, and professionals in both fields need an increased understanding of how the other thinks.

A physician who refers a patient to a mental health professional may have certain ideas about what kind of treatment the patient needs. This seems reasonable, as physicians often have known patients for months or years prior to referring for mental health treatment. However, because of the nature of medical relationships, physicians may not always be clear regarding the mental health needs of patients. For example, I once received a referral from a physician of a patient who had fibromyalgia. He left me a voice mail message indicating that he had given the patient my name and said that he felt the patient needed cognitive-behavioral therapy (CBT). I was aware that much of the medical research on fibromyalgia suggests that CBT is the treatment of choice for these patients. Yet the patient was not interested in CBT and had a number of issues that the physician was unaware of, which warranted another treatment approach. CBT is an intervention that many physicians are aware of, in large part because it has been extensively studied and has been found to have efficacy with a variety of mental health problems. What many physicians may not know, however, is that considerable controversy exists within the field of psychology regarding this research and the related issue of evidence-based therapy. For example, though the research on CBT involves patients with only one Axis I disorder (such as depression), less than 20 percent of all mental health patients have only one, clearly definable Axis I disorder.[1] Many patients have co-morbid Axis I disorders, and many patients also have traits of personality disorders or meet criteria for Axis II disorders, which makes it difficult to generalize about the CBT research. Further, CBT is a very active treatment that requires a great deal of discipline and

when and how to talk to patients about a referral for mental health treatment; this will be addressed in the next sections.

WHEN TO REFER

Although the medical literature suggests that primary care providers engage in routine screening for mental health problems, it is not realistic to expect that physicians can routinely screen every patient in most medical practices. Especially early in the patient–physician relationship, more acute medical issues may need to be addressed. Additionally, because of the sensitive nature of talking about mental health, a referral to a mental health professional is likely to be more successful when it takes place in the context of an established physician–patient relationship of trust. Sometimes it is obvious when a patient needs a referral to a mental health specialist. Such cases include:

1. Patients who are on multiple psychiatric medications or who have not responded to trials of a medication (such as an antidepressant) and who need a referral to a psychiatrist or other professional who specializes in psychotropic medication
2. Patients who are suicidal
3. Patients with multiple psychosocial problems who articulate a need for someone to talk to
4. Patients who need help adjusting to an acute or chronic medical illness
5. Patients with multiple psychosomatic complaints without evidence of physical cause

6. Patients who are actively looking for a therapist and trust the opinion of their primary care physician
7. Patients who need behavioral medicine services such as smoking cessation, stress management, or weight loss

These are the most common kinds of referrals I see. However, some patients may need a referral for psychotherapy based on their physician's opinion that they are having trouble coping, are abusing medications (i.e., benzodiazepines or narcotics), are noncompliant, or may have some underlying and yet undetected psychological problem (such as a personality disorder) that the physician wants to be evaluated. Physicians also refer patients for therapy when they detect the presence of an Axis I disorder such as depression or an anxiety disorder.

It is important to remember that just because a patient may be deemed to need mental health treatment, that doesn't mean that he wants psychological treatment. I often hear from patients and physicians that the process of referring for mental health treatment can take a long time due to patient resistance. Patients are resistant to therapy for a number of reasons. First, therapy and/or psychiatric treatment are expensive. Many patients simply cannot afford it. Patients with HMOs are limited to in-network therapists; often these therapists do not have openings. For patients with complicated medical backgrounds, it is useful for the therapist to have an understanding of medical issues; some therapists do not have this experience, thus making the pool of available professionals smaller. Second, for patients who are seriously ill and going to the doctor frequently, seeing a therapist can feel like going to yet another doctor's appointment; many do not feel they have the time or the energy to do this. Third for patients who are ill, therapy is often viewed as an elective option. This point reflects a widely held view of in our culture that therapy is a luxury, not a necessity. Fourth, a referral to therapy can be experienced by patients as a kind of defeat, indicating that they are not strong enough to manage on their own and exposing their inherent weakness. Finally, patients who have had previous mental health experiences that have been negative often believe that therapy cannot help them. All of these reasons make it difficult for physicians to successfully refer patients to therapy. Timing is a key issue, as of knowing how to talk to patients about such referrals.

Referring a patient specifically for medication evaluation and management is somewhat different than referring for therapy. When to refer for help with psychotropic medication is an individual decision that is based on the physician's comfort level

..., ... unstable or if their disease is active (e.g., active hallucinations, frequent manic episodes). For patients with complicated medication backgrounds who are dependent on narcotics or benzodiazepines, it can be helpful to get the opinion of mental health prescribers who specialize in issues of medication withdrawal. In general, suicidal patients are probably better served by psychiatrists who have experience with medication management in this population and who have admitting privileges to hospitals.

Although so far I have been discussing referrals to individual practitioners, referring patients to support groups is a common practice, especially for patients who have chronic medical illnesses. Support groups are often less threatening to patients, and they provide an opportunity for patients to hear how others are coping with illness; they also offer a forum to gain valuable health-related information. Many patients with medical illnesses express that they feel better after going to a support group because they realize that their situation is not as bad as others. Although this fact is comforting for some patients, others can become more anxious after attending a support group. Some people report that support groups cause them to worry about what could happen to them, for example, if they see patients who have a more serious or advanced form of the same disease. Thus, patients need to make their own decision regarding whether a support group is right for them. Another potential concern is that many support groups are led by paraprofessionals or by peers with the same illness as the group participants. The advantage to this scenario is that patients may feel comfortable describing their illness to someone who knows first-hand what the patient is going through. The disadvantage to groups led by peers or paraprofessionals is that if group dynamics become complicated or if patients have significant psychological problems, the leader may not be qualified to address these issues. Nevertheless, support groups and peer support models are useful for some patients and can be offered to patients in addition to a referral for psychotherapy. Many national organizations offer information, advocacy, and referrals to support groups. Table 1 lists national organizations for those with a variety of disorders; many of these organizations offer referral services, phone counseling, and information on local support groups. Readers wanting more information should contact specific organizations to inquire about resources and support groups in specific areas.

Table 1. National organizations offering services and support groups for medical patients

American Brain Tumor Association (ABTA) 2720 River Road Des Plaines, IL 60018 Telephone: 800–886–2282 E-mail: info@abta.org Internet Web site: http://www.abta.org	**Alzheimer's Association National Office** 225 N. Michigan Ave., Fl. 17 Chicago, IL 60601 Telephone: 800.272.3900 Internet Web site: http://www.alz.org
American Cancer Society (ACS) 1599 Clifton Road, NE. Atlanta, GA 30329–4251 Telephone: 800–227–2345 Internet Web site: http://www.cancer.org	**Crohn's & Colitis Foundation of America** 386 Park Avenue South, 17th floor New York, NY 10016–8804 Phone: 800–932–2423 or 212–685–3440 Fax: 212–779–4098 Email: info@ccfa.org Internet Web site: www.ccfa.org
American Heart Association 7272 Greenville Avenue Dallas, TX 75231 Telephone: 800-242-8721 Internet Web site: http://www.americanheart.org	**American Liver Foundation** 75 Maiden Lane, Suite 603 New York, NY 10038 Telephone: 800–465–4837 Email: info@liverfoundation.org Internet Web site: www.liverfoundation.org
American Stroke Association 7272 Greenville Avenue Dallas TX 75231 Telephone: 888-478-7653 Internet Web site: http://www.americanheart.org	**American Urological Association** 1000 Corporate Boulevard Suite 410 Linthicum, MD 21090 Telephone: 800–828–7866 Internet Web site: http://www.afud.org

The Brain Tumor Society
124 Watertown Street, Suite 3–H
Watertown, MA 02472
Telephone: 800–770–8287

Internet Web site: http://www.
cancercare.org

Cancer Hope Network
Two North Road
Chester, NJ 07930
Telephone: 877–467–3638
E-mail: info@cancerhopenetwork.org
Internet Web site: http://www.
cancerhopenetwork.org

Colon Cancer Alliance (CCA)
175 Ninth Avenue
New York, NY 10011
Telephone: 877–422–2030
E-mail: info@ccalliance.org
Internet Web site: http://www.
ccalliance.org

Colorectal Cancer Network
P. O. Box 182
Kensington, MD 20895–0182
Telephone: 301–879–1500
E-mail: ccnetwork@colorectal-
cancer.net
Internet Web site: http://www.
colorectal-cancer.net

Fertile Hope
P. O. Box 624
New York, NY 10014
Telephone: 888–994–4673
(888–994–HOPE)

E-mail: lbeck@fertilehope.org
Internet Web site: http://www.
fertilehope.org

Hospice Link
Three Unity Square
P. O. Box 98
Machiasport, ME 04655–0098
Telephone: 800–331–1620
E-mail: HOSPICEALL@aol.com
Internet Web site: http://www.
hospiceworld.org

**International Myeloma Foundation
(IMF)**
12650 Riverside Drive, Suite 206
North Hollywood, CA 91607–3421
Telephone: 800–452–2873
(800–452–CURE)
E-mail: TheIMF@myeloma.org
Internet Web site:
http://www.myeloma.org

Kidney Cancer Association
1234 Sherman Avenue, Suite 203
Evanston, IL 60202–1375
Telephone: 800–850–9132
E-mail: office@curekidneycancer.org
Internet Web site: http://www.
curekidneycancer.org

Lance Armstrong Foundation (LAF)
P. O. Box 161150
Austin, TX 78716
Telephone: 512-236-8820
Internet Web site: http://www.laf.org

(Continued)

Table 1. (*Continued*)

The Leukemia and Lymphoma Society 1311 Mamaroneck Avenue White Plains, NY 10605–5221 Telephone: 800–955–4572 E-mail: infocenter@leukemia-lymphoma.org Internet Web site: http://www.leukemia-lymphoma.org	**National Bone Marrow Transplant Link** 20411 West 12 Mile Road, Suite 108 Southfield, MI 48076 Telephone: 800–546–5268 E-mail: nbmtlink@aol.com Internet Web site: http://www.nbmtlink.org/
Living Beyond Breast Cancer (LBBC) 10 East Athens Avenue, Suite 204 Ardmore, PA 19003 Telephone: 888–753–5222 E-mail: mail@lbbc.org Internet Web site: http://www.lbbc.org	**National Breast Cancer Coalition (NBCC)** 1101 17th Street, NW, Suite 1300 Washington, DC 20036 Telephone: 800–622–2838 E-mail: info@stopbreastcancer.org Internet Web site: http://www.stopbreastcancer.org
The Lung Cancer Alliance (LCA) 888 16th Street, NW, Suite 800 Washington, DC 20006 Telephone: 800–298–2436 E-mail: info@lungcanceralliance.org Internet Web site: http://www.lungcanceralliance.org	**National Coalition for Cancer Survivorship (NCCS)** 1010 Wayne Avenue, Suite 770 Silver Spring, MD 20910–5600 Telephone: 877–622–7937 E-mail: info@canceradvocacy.org Internet Web site: http://www.canceradvocacy.org
The Lustgarten Foundation for Pancreatic Cancer Research 1111 Stewart Avenue Bethpage, NY 11714 Telephone: 866–789–1000 E-mail: Available through the Web site Internet Web site: http://www.lustgartenfoundation.org	**National Fibromyalgia Association** 2200 Glassell Street, Suite A Orange, CA 92865 Phone: (714) 921-0150 Internet Web site: http://www.fmaware.org
National Asian Women's Health Organization (NAWHO) 250 Montgomery Street, Suite 900 San Francisco, CA 94104 Telephone: 415–989–9747 E-mail: nawho@nawho.org Internet Web site: http://www.nawho.org	**National Hospice and Palliative Care Organization (NHPCO)** 1700 Diagonal Road, Suite 625 Alexandria, VA 22314 Telephone: 800–658–8898 E-mail: info@nhpco.org Internet Web site: http://www.nhpco.org

National Ovarian Cancer Coalition (NOCC)
500 Northeast Spanish River
Boulevard, Suite 14

Newport Beach, CA 92663
Telephone: 949-646-8000
E-mail:
info@oralcancerfoundation.org
Internet Web site: http://www.
oralcancerfoundation.org

Parkinson's Disease Foundation
1359 Broadway, Suite 1509
New York, NY 10018
Telephone: 212.923.4700
Email: info@pdf.org
Web site: www.pdf.org

Prostate Cancer Foundation
1250 Fourth Street
Santa Monica, CA 90401
Telephone: 800–757–2873
E-mail: info@prostatecancer
foundation.org
Internet Web site: http://www.
prostatecancerfoundation.org/

Support for People with Oral and Head and Neck Cancer (SPOHNC)
Post Office Box 53
Locust Valley, NY 11560–0053

Telephone: 800–377–0928
E-mail: info@spohnc.org
Internet Web site:
http://www.spohnc.org

breastcancerinfo.com

Thyroid Cancer Survivors' Association, Inc.
Post Office Box 1545
New York, NY 10159–1545
Telephone: 877–588–7904
E-mail: thyca@thyca.org
Internet Web site:
http://www.thyca.org

United Ostomy Association, Inc.
19772 MacArthur Boulevard,
Suite 200
Irvine, CA 92612–2405
Phone: 800–826–0826 or
949–660–8624
Fax: 949–660–9262
Email: info@uoa.org
Internet Web site: www.uoa.org

HOW TO REFER

Unless a patient requests a referral to a mental health provider, it can be difficult for physicians to know how to talk to patients about mental health referrals. Many patients do not want to see a mental health professional. Some patients prefer the comfort of the relationship with their primary care physician and would prefer to maintain the physician as a confidante. Other patients are afraid of talking about their thoughts and feelings because of a fear of being overwhelmed. Patients who get the message that the physician has nothing left to offer can feel resentful. Additionally, patients who are fearful of being abandoned often worry that a referral to a mental health professional indicates that they are being "fired" by the physician. Thus, a key point in referring patients to mental health therapists is to communicate that they referral does not indicate abandonment. This is especially important for patients who have borderline personality dynamics and/or those who are likely to feel abandoned. The message that is most helpful to communicate to patients in these situations is that they are not being abandoned but that the referral indicates that the physician wants them to get extra support. This is a good strategy for all patients. One physician recently told me that she tells patients that she wants to refer for mental health consultation not because she doesn't want to help her patients but because her expertise lies in the patient's physical health and that someone else better qualified can help to take care of their mental health.

Another common difficulty with referring for mental health treatment occurs when patients have psychological problems that appear to be exacerbating or causing their physical symptoms. Such patients often worry that they will be told that their symptoms are "all in their mind." In such cases, it is often helpful to reinforce to patients that though their physical problems are real, psychological factors can make physical problems worse. Since patients often wonder how this can be so, I often tell them that the physical consequences of stress, anxiety, and depression increase the perception of pain and can cause other physiological changes that impact health. I also point out that everyone experiences physiological changes as a result of stress and emotions, but that persons who are already ill may be more vulnerable to the impact of these changes. Such an approach often helps patients to feel less defensive about the cause of their symptoms and normalizes the physical impact of psychological issues.

Especially since mental health treatment is stigmatized, patients often need education regarding the process of therapy and mental health services. If patients are worried that seeing a mental health professional indicates that they ~~...~~

~~...~~ patients lives, and as someone with whom they can discuss the psychological implications of medical illness. This last point is important because many patients do not feel that they can talk about medical problems and their impact with a therapist. Patients often have the misconception that going to see a mental health clinician means that they must discuss their childhood and that they have to discuss in detail painful experiences from their background. This is not the case; if patients are concerned about this, this myth should be dispelled. Although certainly most mental health professionals would agree that early developmental factors play a role in a patient's psychological development, these do not need to be discussed in excruciating detail as part of contemporary mental health treatment. For practitioners who do use a psychoanalytic approach (including myself), issues related to early developmental factors can be addressed indirectly though discussing the impact of these issues on current relationships if the therapist and the patient agree that it may be useful to do so.

Other strategies in referring patients for mental health services include telling patients that they should meet with the mental health professional once to see what they think. Many physicians provide two or three names of mental health professionals and encourage patients to interview each until they find a therapist that is a good fit. This not only helps patients to feel empowered in choosing their own clinician, but also helps to allay the common fear that therapy is a never-ending process and that one visit means that they are committing to being in treatment for years. Also, the success of psychotherapy is highly dependent on the personality match of the patient and the therapist. In fact, most psychotherapy research suggests that the outcome of psychotherapy is attributable to "nonspecific" factors and one of these factors may be the personality fit between patient and therapist.

Some physicians prefer to call mental health therapists to tell them that they have referred a patient. In my practice, I prefer that the physician provides a quick summary of major medical problems as well as concerns about a patient's mental health. If a physician wants me to follow up with him or her regarding my diagnosis and treatment decisions, it is helpful to know that as well. Some mental health providers do write a consult note to give to the physician (as is the case among medical specialties), but not all therapists do this routinely. If the physician wants an opinion on whether an antidepressant should be used to treat the patient and which medication is recommended, it is important to communicate this. Sometimes physicians refer patients for therapy and think that an antidepressant would not be helpful or would interact with medications the patient is taking. This is important to communicate as some patients see a mental health referral solely as a route to obtaining medication. If physicians believe that a trial of therapy should precede thinking about medication (which is a valid option for some depression and anxiety disorders), it is important to communicate this as well. Especially for complicated patients, collaboration between therapists and physicians is important; in reality, such collaboration doesn't take place until an acute medical or psychological issue arises. Therefore, it is often helpful for physicians to specify to the mental health clinician what kind of follow-up they prefer.

CONCLUSIONS

Referring to a mental health professional can be complicated, but is a common and necessary part of practicing medicine. Since what physicians can offer is often concrete, immediate, and practical, it is understandable that patients may have trouble appreciating the need for mental health services, as these services may not offer the same tangible benefits. Additionally, because the philosophical differences between medicine and psychology reflect the idea that the mind and the body function separately, it can be hard for patients to see that psychotherapy can be useful to them. However, as we saw in Chapter 1, the mind and the body are intimately connected and emotional states contribute to physical health and disease. This is perhaps the most compelling reason to refer medical patients for psychotherapy. Given the serious consequences of depression and anxiety on health, treating these emotional problems may potentially ward off future

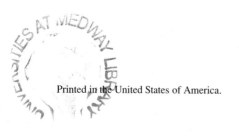